PREFIXES AND SUFFIXES

MEDICAL TERMINOLOGY

The Big Book of Medical Terminology Workbook

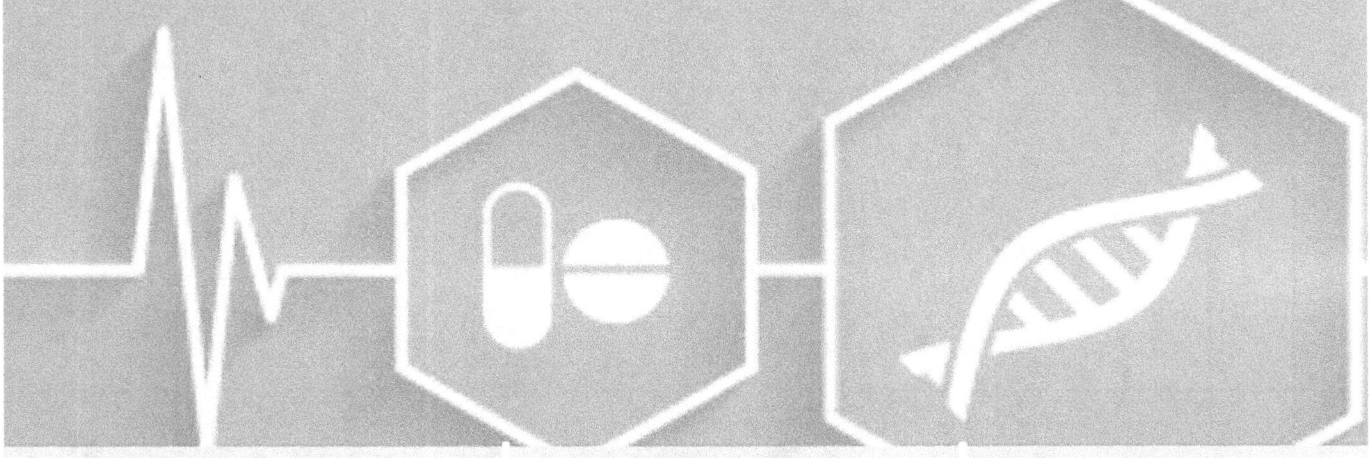

473+ Terms	Prefixes	Suffixes
Matching Game	Table Review	Word Search
Crosswords	Quiz	Test

PREFIXES & SUFFIXES -

Medical Terminology Table Review

Medical Terminology

Prefix/Suffix	Meaning
a-	without or lack of
ab-	away (away from)
abdomin/o-	belly
-able	capable of
abort/io	to miscarry or miscarrying (natural or induced)
abrupt/io-	to tear away from
abcess	a going away
-ac	refers to or pertains to
-ory	refers to or pertains to
-us	refers to or pertains to
acanth/o-	thorny (skin growth)
access/o-	supplemental
acetabul/o-	vinegar cup or hip joint (for femur)
acne	pointed
acoust/i-	hearing
acr/o-	extremities, height and pointed
acrom/i-	extremities, height and pointed
actin/o-	sun, ray, radium
acu-	sharp
acus-	sharp
ad-	near or beside
aden/o-	gland
adhes/io-	to stick (together)
adip/o-	fat
aer/o-	air or gas
af-	toward
-age	relates to or pertains to
aggglutnin/o-	to clump
-agogue	inducing or leading
-agon	walls
-agra	pain
-al	refers to
alb/o-	white
albumin/o-	egg white
alges/i-	pain
-algia	pain
alimento/o	to nourish
alopec/i-	fox mange or baldness
alveol/i-	cavity
ambi-	both
amblyo-	dull

ambul/o-	to walk
-amine	nitrogen compound
amino-	organic compound
amnesi/o-	forgetful
amnio-	lambs caul 'small cap'
amphi-	both
amylo-	starch
an-	lack of or without
an/o-	ring
ana-	apart or up
ancone-	elbow
andr/o-	man or male
anecto-	without expansion or dilation
angi/o-	vessel
angin/o-	to choke
anil/i-	old women
anis/o-	unequal
ankyl/o-	fuse or bind
anomal/y	abnormal
ante-	before
anter/o-	before or foremost (in front)
anthr/o-	coal or carbuncle
anthrac/o-	coal or carbuncle
anthrop/o-	human
anti-	against
antr/o-	cavity
antr/um-	cavity or cavern
anuerysm-	dilation or ballooning
anxio-	restlessness, uneasy, apprehensive
-apheresis	to remove or separate
apo-	above or upon
aponeur/o-	upon tendon (sheet or sheath around tendon)
append/o-	appendage
aqua-	water
-ar	refers to
ar-	without or lack of
acrachn/	spider
arachino-	spider
arche/o-	first
arche-	first
-aria	air
arteri/o-	artery
arthr/o-	joint
articul/o-	jointed
-ary	refers to
asbest/o-	unquenchable

ascar/i-	worm
asco-	bag
-ase	enzyme
aspergill/o-	to sprinkle
aster/o-	star
-asthenia	weakness
asthma-	panting
-ate	refers to or action
atelo-	incomplete, without end, imperfect (ending)
athero-	porridge or yellow fat
-ation	process of or procedure of
-ition	process of or procedure of
atm/o-	vapor or steam
-artresia	closure
atri/o-	chamber
attrit/i-	wearing out
audi-	hearing
aur/i-	ear
auricul/o-	ear
auscult/o-	to listen
auto-	self
aut-	self
avuls/i-	to tear
axill/o-	armpit or central
axio-	axle or axis
axo-	axle or axis
azoto-	urea nitrogen
azygo-	single
Bacill/o	ROD-LIKE
Bacteri/o-	ROD
Balan/o-	PENIS (GLANS PENIS)
Baro-	WEIGHT
Bary-	HEAVY
Bas/o-	basic
Bas/io-	at a base
Bene-	good or normal
Benign/i-	kind
Beri-	weakness
Bi-	two
Bil/i- (bil-)	bile or gall
Bin-	two
bio-	life
-blast	beginning or young
bleb/o- (bulla-)	blister
blenno-	mucus
blepharo- (palpebro-)	eyelid

bol/o-	lump or ball
-borg	orgasm
brach/i-	arm
brachy-	short
brady-	slow
brevi-	short
bronch/i-	windpipe or tracea-like
brux-	grinding
brucca-	cheek
bulba-	bister or vesicle
bula-	blister or vesicle
bulimo-	hunger
burs/o-	sac, wine-sac, or pouch
cac/o-	diseased or bad
cal/o-	heat, heated or hot
calcane/o-	heel
calcin/o-	calcium
calco-	pebbles or granules (of calcium mineral)
caligi/o-	dim vision
calyx-	cups
calix-	cups
call/o-	hardened skin
calx-	heel or lime
candid/i-	glowing white
canth/o-	corner of eye
capill/o-	hair-like
capit/o-	head
capn/o-	carbon dioxide
capsulo-	little box
caput-	head
carb/o-	carbon atoms, coal, or charcoal
carbun/o-	glowing ember
carbuncul/o-	glowing ember
carcin/o-	crab-like
cardi/o-	heart
carp/o-	wrist
cata-	breakdown or down
cataract	waterfall or cloudiness
catarrh-	to flow down
catheter/o-	to let down into
caud/o-	tall or toward tall
caust/o-	burn or heat
cau-	burn or heat
caus-	burn or heat
cav-	hollow
cebo-	meal or food

cec/o-	blind pouch
-cece	navel
-cele	swelling or tumor
cell/o-	abdomen or belly
cellul/o-	chambers
cement/o-	hard
ceno-	empty or common
keno-	empty or common
-centesis	surgical puncture to drain fluid
centi-	one-hundredth apart
centr/i-	center
centro-	center
cephalo-	head
-cept-	receiver
cerbr/o-	brain
ceru-	wax
cerv/i-	neck
chalas/i-	relaxation
chalaz/io-	hailstone (eyelid sebaceous cyst)
chancr/o-	ulcer (sore)
cheil/o-	lip
chilo-	lip
chiasma	a crossing
chiro-	hand
chlamyd/i-	to cloak or cover
chlor/o-	green
cholangio-	bile duct
chole-	bile or gall (ingredient of)
cholecyst/o-	gallbladder
choledoch/o-	gallbladder duct (canal)
cholera-	billary acute diarrhea
chondr/o-	cartilage
chordo- (cordo-)	cord
chorea-	dancing (shaking)
chrom/o-	colored
chyme-	juice
chyle-	juice
-cicatrix	scar
-cid	to kill
cil/i-	eyelash-like
cili-	eyelash or eyelash like
cimex-	bug
cine/o-	movement filming
circum-	around
cirrh/o-	yellow-oranged (jaundiced)
-cis	cut or to cut

cistern/o-	cavity
-clalasia	relaxation
-clast	breakdown
-clas	breakdown
clavicul/o-	collar bone (little key shape)
cleido-	hook, clavicle or collar bone
clino-	bent
clon/o-	turmoil
clubb/o-	rounding
-clysis	irrigation or injection
co-	two
coagulo/o-	clotting or clot
-coccus	berry
coccyg/o-	tailbone
cochle/o-	snail-like
coel-	hollow belly (cavity)
coit/o-	to come together (sexual union; inter/course "between/a flowing")
col/o-	colon big or large intestine
colon/o-	colon big or large intestine
colla/o-	glue
-collis	twisted
colob/o-	to mutilate
colpo-	vagina
com-	together
comato-	deep sleep
con-	together
conch/a-	shell
concuss/i-	violent shaking
condyl/o-	knuckle (nob)
coni/o-	dust
-conis	cone shaped
conjuctiv/o-	together joined (united)
-continence	contained
contra-	against
contrecoup	counter blow
contus/i-	bruise
convolo-	to roll together
corac/o-	crows beak (shape)
cord-	vocal chords cord
core/o-	pupil or iris (rainbow)
cori/o-	skin
corne/o-	cornea or horn (shape)
cornu-	horn or horny
coron/o-	crowning
coronal plane (aka: frontal plane)	crowning frontal body cut
corp/o-	body

cortic/o-	bark, outer bark, rind, or cortex
cost/o-	rib
cox/a-	hip, hip joint, (pelvis and femur)
cox/o-	hip, hip joint, (pelvis and femur)
crani/o-	skull
cras/o-	mixture
-creas	fleshy or flesh
crenat/o-	notched
cric/o-	ring
-crine	secrete
-crin	secrete
-crit	separate
cruc/i-	cross or cross-like
crur/o-	leg thigh or femur
crus/o-	leg thigh or femur
crust/-	scab or outer coat
cryo-	cold
crypto-	secret
cub/o-	cube or cube shaped
cubit/o-	elbow
culd/o-	blind pouch
-cule	little
cune/i-	wedge
currett/o-	scooping or scraping
-cusis	hearing
cusp/i-	pointed
cuti/o- (cut-)	skin
cutis-	skin
cyan/o-	blue
cycl/o-	circle
-cyesis	pregnancy
cyst/o-	bladder or sac
cyst-	bladder or sac
cyst/i-	bladder or sac
cystido-	bladder or sac
cyte-	cell or chamber
cyt-	cell or chamber
cyth-	cell or chamber
-cytosis	increase (in number)
dacryo-	tear
dactylo-	digits (fingers and toes)
de-	away
debride-	removal
deca-	one/tenth (1/10)
decem-	one/tenth (1/10)
decub/o-	to lie down

deep	most inward
deka-, dek-	ten
delta	fan shaped or triangular
dem/o-	people
demi-	half
dendr/o-	tree-shaped
DENT/O-	TOOTH OR TEETH
DON'T/O-	TOOTH OR TEETH
DEPRESS-	LOWER
DERM/O-	SKIN
DERMAT/O-	SKIN
-DESIS	BINDING, TO BAND OR A BAND
desmo-	ligament (also tendon)
deuter/o-	second or secondary
dextr/o-	rght
di-	two
dia-	across, through, total or complete, or between
diaphoro-	excessive sweating
-didymis	testis or teste
different-	to separate or apart
-deferens	to separate or apart
digit-	finger or toe
diplo-	double or two
dips/o-	thirst or thirsty
dipther/i-	membrane
dis-	away from or reversed
dist/o-	farther from
diverticul/o-	outpouching
doch/o-	duct or canal
doct/o-	to teach or teacher
dol/o-	pain
dolich/o-	long, seperation, dislocation
dors/o-	back
dos/e- (dose)	a giving
-dote	what is given
dracuncul/o-	little dragon (worm)
dromo-	running
du/o-	two
duct/o-	to draw or to lead (motion) away
duoden/o-	twelve
dura-	hard
dwarf/o-	small
dy/o-	two or a pair
dynam/o-	work or strength
-dynia	pain
dys-	diffucult, faulty or painful

-e	instrument
e-	out or remove
-eal	refers to
ec-	outside, outward, outer or out
ect-	outside, outward, outer or out
ecto-	outside, outward, outer or out
ecchymo/-	juice out
eccrine-	secreting or to secrete
echin/o-	prickly, spiny or notched
echo-	sound
-ectasis	dilation
-estasy	dilation
-ectomy	excisio or removal
eczema	to boil out
edema-	swelling
ef-	away or out
effer-	away or out
effus-	away or out
electr/o-	electrical
-ellum	lesser or smaller
em-	in
emac/i-	to grow thin
embryo-	early
-emesis	vomit
ernia	blood
emmetr/o-	normal or correct
emphysema	puffed up
en-	in
enamel	hard
encephal/o-	within head brain
-enchyma	anything poured in (essential organ part)
endo-	within or inside
enema	injection
entero-	intestine (usually refers to small intestine)
enuresis-	to void (expel) urine
eosin/o-	rose red (color)
epi-	upon
episi/o-	pubic region
-er	one who
-or	one who
-ergo	work or labor
eruct/o-	belching
erythermat/o-	red or flushed
erthr/o-	red
eschar	scab
eso-	toward

esthes/i-	feeling (physical)
estr/o-	female
ethm/o-	sieve
eti/o-	cause
eti/o-	cause
eu-	good or normal
ex-	out, outside, outward
exo-	out, outside, outward
extra-	out, outside, outward
facet	face
fac-	face
faci/o-	face
-facient	making
fasc/i-	band
febr/o-	fever
fec/o-	stool, fecal matter, or dung
scato-	stool, fecal matter, or dung
sterco-	srool, fecal matter or dung
femor/o-	thigh
fenestr/o-	window
-ference	to carry
ferro-	iron
fet/o-	young
fibrill/o-	to quiver
fibrin/o-	fiber-like
fibro-	fiber
fibul/o-	to clasp
fil-	thread
fila-	thread
fili-	thread
filar/i-	thread
fimbri/o-	fingers
fiss-	to split or splitting
fistul/o-	pipe or pipe-stem
flacci/o-	soft
flagell/o-	whip
flat/o-	to blow
flex-	to bend
-flect	to bend
flu-	flowing
-flux	to flow
foc/o-	center or hearth
fontan/o-	little fountain
formamen/o-	opening
fore-	before
-form	shaped shape or form

fossa-	furrow or shallow depression
fract/o-	to break
front/o-	forehead or before
-fuge	to flee
fulgur/o-	to lighten (with sparks burning tissue)
fulv/o-	brown
fund/o-	base or lage part (organ body)
fungi-	mushroom
furc/o-	branch or fork
furun/o-	boil
galact/o-	milk
gamet/o-	to marry, unite, or sexual union
gam/o-	to marry, unite, or sexual union
gangli/o-	knot swelling or collection knot
gangren/o-	eating sore
gastr/o-	stomach
gelat/o-	freeze or congeal
gelatino-	freeze or congeal

PREFIXES & SUFFIXES -

Medical Terminology Flash Cards

Terms on ODD pages and Definitions on EVEN pages

a-	-able
ab-	abort/io
abdomin/o-	abrupt/io-
-ac	abcess

capable of	without or lack of
to miscarry or miscarrying (natural or induced)	away (away from)
to tear away from	belly
a going away	refers to or pertains to

-ory	access/o-
-us	acetabul/o-
acanth/o-	acne
acr/o-	acoust/i-

supplemental	refers to or pertains to
vinegar cup or hip joint (for femur)	refers to or pertains to
pointed	thorny (skin growth)
hearing	extremities, height and pointed

acrom/i-	acus-
actin/o-	ad-
acu-	aden/o-
adip/o-	adhes/io-

sharp	extremities, height and pointed
near or beside	sun, ray, radium
gland	sharp
to stick (together)	fat

aer/o-	aggglutnin/o-
af-	-agogue
-age	-agon
-al	-agra

to clump	air or gas
inducing or leading	toward
walls	relates to or pertains to
pain	refers to

alb/o-	-algia
albumin/o-	alimento/o
alges/i-	alopec/i-
ambi-	alveol/i-

pain	white
to nourish	egg white
fox mange or baldness	pain
cavity	both

amblyo-	amino-
ambul/o-	amnesi/o-
-amine	amnio-
amylo-	amphi-

organic compound	dull
forgetful	to walk
lambs caul 'small cap'	nitrogen compound
both	starch

an-	ancone-
an/o-	andr/o-
ana-	anecto-
angin/o-	angi/o-

elbow	lack of or without
man or male	ring
without expansion or dilation	apart or up
vessel	to choke

anil/i-	anomal/y
anis/o-	ante-
ankyl/o-	anter/o-
anthrac/o-	anthr/o-

abnormal	old women
before	unequal
before or foremost (in front)	fuse or bind
coal or carbuncle	coal or carbuncle

anthrop/o-	antr/um-
anti-	anuerysm-
antr/o-	anxio-
apo-	-apheresis

cavity or cavern	human
dilation or ballooning	against
restlessness, uneasy, apprehensive	cavity
to remove or separate	above or upon

aponeur/o-	-ar
append/o-	ar-
aqua-	acrachn/
arche/o-	arachino-

refers to	upon tendon (sheet or sheath around tendon)
without or lack of	appendage
spider	water
spider	first

arche-	arthr/o-
-aria	articul/o-
arteri/o-	-ary
ascar/i-	asbest/o-

joint	first
jointed	air
refers to	artery
unquenchable	worm

asco-	aster/o-
-ase	-asthenia
aspergill/o-	asthma-
atelo-	-ate

star	bag
weakness	enzyme
panting	to sprinkle
refers to or action	incomplete, without end, imperfect (ending)

athero-	atm/o-
-ation	-artresia
-ition	atri/o-
audi-	attrit/i-

vapor or steam	porridge or yellow fat
closure	process of or procedure of
chamber	process of or procedure of
wearing out	hearing

aur/i-	auto-
auricul/o-	aut-
auscult/o-	avuls/i-
axio-	axill/o-

self	ear
self	ear
to tear	to listen
armpit or central	axle or axis

axo-	Bacill/o
azoto-	Bacteri/o-
azygo-	Balan/o-
Bary-	Baro-

ROD-LIKE	axle or axis
ROD	urea nitrogen
PENIS (GLANS PENIS)	single
WEIGHT	HEAVY

Bas/o-	Benign/i-
Bas/io-	Beri-
Bene-	Bi-
Bin-	Bil/i- (bil-)

kind	basic
weakness	at a base
two	good or normal
bile or gall	two

bio-	blenno-
-blast	blepharo- (palpebro-)
bleb/o- (bulla-)	bol/o-
brach/i-	-borg

mucus	life
eyelid	beginning or young
lump or ball	blister
orgasm	arm

brachy-	bronch/i-
brady-	brux-
brevi-	brucca-
bula-	bulba-

<table>
<tr><td>windpipe or tracea-like</td><td>short</td></tr>
<tr><td>grinding</td><td>slow</td></tr>
<tr><td>cheek</td><td>short</td></tr>
<tr><td>bister or vesicle</td><td>blister or vesicle</td></tr>
</table>

bulimo-	cal/o-
burs/o-	calcane/o-
cac/o-	calcin/o-
caligi/o-	calco-

heat, heated or hot	hunger
heel	sac, wine-sac, or pouch
calcium	diseased or bad
pebbles or granules (of calcium mineral)	dim vision

calyx-	calx-
calix-	candid/i-
call/o-	canth/o-
capit/o-	capill/o-

heel or lime	cups
glowing white	cups
corner of eye	hardened skin
hair-like	head

capn/o-	carb/o-
capsulo-	carbun/o-
caput-	carbuncul/o-
cardi/o-	carcin/o-

carbon atoms, coal, or charcoal	carbon dioxide
glowing ember	little box
glowing ember	head
crab-like	heart

carp/o-	catarrh-
cata-	catheter/o-
cataract	caud/o-
cau-	caust/o-

to flow down	wrist
to let down into	breakdown or down
tall or toward tall	waterfall or cloudiness
burn or heat	burn or heat

caus-	cec/o-
cav-	-cece
cebo-	-cele
cellul/o-	cell/o-

blind pouch	burn or heat
navel	hollow
swelling or tumor	meal or food
abdomen or belly	chambers

cement/o-	-centesis
ceno-	centi-
keno-	centr/i-
cephalo-	centro-

surgical puncture to drain fluid	hard
one-hundredth apart	empty or common
center	empty or common
center	head

-cept-	cerv/i-
cerbr/o-	chalas/i-
ceru-	chalaz/io-
cheil/o-	chancr/o-

neck	receiver
relaxation	brain
hailstone (eyelid sebaceous cyst)	wax
ulcer (sore)	lip

chilo-	chlamyd/i-
chiasma	chlor/o-
chiro-	cholangio-
cholecyst/o-	chole-

to cloak or cover	lip
green	a crossing
bile duct	hand
bile or gall (ingredient of)	gallbladder

choledoch/o-	chordo- (cordo-)
cholera-	chorea-
chondr/o-	chrom/o-
chyle-	chyme-

cord	gallbladder duct (canal)
dancing (shaking)	billary acute diarrhea
colored	cartilage
juice	juice

-cicatrix	cili-
-cid	cimex-
cil/i-	cine/o-
cirrh/o-	circum-

eyelash or eyelash like	scar
bug	to kill
movement filming	eyelash-like
around	yellow-oranged (jaundiced)

-cis	-clast
cistern/o-	-clas
-clalasia	clavicul/o-
clino-	cleido-

breakdown	cut or to cut
breakdown	cavity
collar bone (little key shape)	relaxation
hook, clavicle or collar bone	bent

clon/o-	co-
clubb/o-	coagulo/o-
-clysis	-coccus
cochle/o-	coccyg/o-

two	turmoil
clotting or clot	rounding
berry	irrigation or injection
tailbone	snail-like

coel-	colon/o-
coit/o-	colla/o-
col/o-	-collis
colpo-	colob/o-

colon big or large intestine	hollow belly (cavity)
glue	to come together (sexual union; inter/course "between/a flowing")
twisted	colon big or large intestine
to mutilate	vagina

com-	conch/a-
comato-	concuss/i-
con-	condyl/o-
-conis	coni/o-

shell	together
violent shaking	deep sleep
knuckle (nob)	together
dust	cone shaped

conjuctiv/o-	contrecoup
-continence	contus/i-
contra-	convolo-
cord-	corac/o-

counter blow	together joined (united)
bruise	contained
to roll together	against
crows beak (shape)	vocal chords cord

core/o-	cornu-
cori/o-	coron/o-
corne/o-	coronal plane (aka: frontal plane)
cortic/o-	corp/o-

horn or horny	pupil or iris (rainbow)
crowning	skin
crowning frontal body cut	cornea or horn (shape)
body	bark, outer bark, rind, or cortex

cost/o-	crani/o-
cox/a-	cras/o-
cox/o-	-creas
cric/o-	crenat/o-

skull	rib
mixture	hip, hip joint, (pelvis and femur)
fleshy or flesh	hip, hip joint, (pelvis and femur)
notched	ring

-crine	cruc/i-
-crin	crur/o-
-crit	crus/o-
cryo-	crust/-

cross or cross-like	secrete
leg thigh or femur	secrete
leg thigh or femur	separate
scab or outer coat	cold

crypto-	culd/o-
cub/o-	-cule
cubit/o-	cune/i-
-cusis	currett/o-

blind pouch	secret
little	cube or cube shaped
wedge	elbow
scooping or scraping	hearing

cusp/i-	cyan/o-
cuti/o- (cut-)	cycl/o-
cutis-	-cyesis
cyst-	cyst/o-

blue	pointed
circle	skin
pregnancy	skin
bladder or sac	bladder or sac

cyst/i-	cyt-
cystido-	cyth-
cyte-	-cytosis
dactylo-	dacryo-

cell or chamber	bladder or sac
cell or chamber	bladder or sac
increase (in number)	cell or chamber
tear	digits (fingers and toes)

de-	decem-
debride-	decub/o-
deca-	deep
delta	deka-, dek-

one/tenth (1/10)	away
to lie down	removal
most inward	one/tenth (1/10)
ten	fan shaped or triangular

dem/o-	DENT/O-
demi-	DON'T/O-
dendr/o-	DEPRESS-
DERMAT/O-	DERM/O-

TOOTH OR TEETH	people
TOOTH OR TEETH	half
LOWER	tree-shaped
SKIN	SKIN

-DESIS	dextr/o-
desmo-	di-
deuter/o-	dia-
-didymis	diaphoro-

rght	**BINDING, TO BAND OR A BAND**
two	ligament (also tendon)
across, through, total or complete, or between	second or secondary
excessive sweating	testis or teste

different-	diplo-
-deferens	dips/o-
digit-	dipther/i-
dist/o-	dis-

<table>
<tr><td>double or two</td><td>to separate or apart</td></tr>
<tr><td>thirst or thirsty</td><td>to separate or apart</td></tr>
<tr><td>membrane</td><td>finger or toe</td></tr>
<tr><td>away from or reversed</td><td>farther from</td></tr>
</table>

diverticul/o-	dol/o-
doch/o-	dolich/o-
doct/o-	dors/o-
-dote	dos/e- (dose)

pain	outpouching
long, seperation, dislocation	duct or canal
back	to teach or teacher
a giving	what is given

dracuncul/o-	duct/o-
dromo-	duoden/o-
du/o-	dura-
dy/o-	dwarf/o-

to draw or to lead (motion) away	little dragon (worm)
twelve	running
hard	two
small	two or a pair

dynam/o-	-e
-dynia	e-
dys-	-eal
ect-	ec-

instrument	work or strength
out or remove	pain
refers to	diffucult, faulty or painful
outside, outward, outer or out	outside, outward, outer or out

ecto-	echin/o-
ecchymo/-	echo-
eccrine-	-ectasis
-ectomy	-estasy

prickly, spiny or notched	outside, outward, outer or out
sound	juice out
dilation	secreting or to secrete
dilation	excisio or removal

eczema	effer-
edema-	effus-
ef-	electr/o-
em-	-ellum

away or out	to boil out
away or out	swelling
electrical	away or out
lesser or smaller	in

emac/i-	ernia
embryo-	emmetr/o-
-emesis	emphysema
enamel	en-

blood	to grow thin
normal or correct	early
puffed up	vomit
in	hard

encephal/o-	enema
-enchyma	entero-
endo-	enuresis-
epi-	eosin/o-

injection	within head brain
intestine (usually refers to small intestine)	anything poured in (essential organ part)
to void (expel) urine	within or inside
rose red (color)	upon

episi/o-	-ergo
-er	eruct/o-
-or	erythermat/o-
eschar	erthr/o-

work or labor	pubic region
belching	one who
red or flushed	one who
red	scab

eso-	ethm/o-
esthes/i-	eti/o-
estr/o-	eti/o-
ex-	eu-

sieve	toward
cause	feeling (physical)
cause	female
good or normal	out, outside, outward

exo-	fac-
extra-	faci/o-
facet	-facient
febr/o-	fasc/i-

face	out, outside, outward
face	out, outside, outward
making	face
band	fever

fec/o-	femor/o-
scato-	fenestr/o-
sterco-	-ference
fet/o-	ferro-

thigh	stool, fecal matter, or dung
window	stool, fecal matter, or dung
to carry	srool, fecal matter or dung
iron	young

fibrill/o-	fibul/o-
fibrin/o-	fil-
fibro-	fila-
filar/i-	fili-

to clasp	to quiver
thread	fiber-like
thread	fiber
thread	thread

fimbri/o-	flacci/o-
fiss-	flagell/o-
fistul/o-	flat/o-
-flect	flex-

soft	fingers
whip	to split or splitting
to blow	pipe or pipe-stem
to bend	to bend

flu-	fontan/o-
-flux	formamen/o-
foc/o-	fore-
fossa-	-form

little fountain	flowing
opening	to flow
before	center or hearth
shaped shape or form	furrow or shallow depression

fract/o-	fulgur/o-
front/o-	fulv/o-
-fuge	fund/o-
furc/o-	fungi-

to lighten (with sparks burning tissue)	to break
brown	forehead or before
base or lage part (organ body)	to flee
mushroom	branch or fork

furun/o-	gam/o-
galact/o-	gangli/o-
gamet/o-	gangren/o-
gelat/o-	gastr/o-

to marry, unite, or sexual union	boil
knot swelling or collection knot	milk
eating sore	to marry, unite, or sexual union
stomach	freeze or congeal

gelatinofreeze or congeal

PREFIXES & SUFFIXES -

Medical Terminology Bingo Game

B I N G O

B	I	N	G	O
-ectasis	Bacteri/o-	fili-	-er	calix-
fontan/o-	cau-	chalaz/io-	brucca-	access/o-
-flect	-clalasia	FREE	dors/o-	cord-
foc/o-	aer/o-	e-	extra-	albumin/o-
axill/o-	colla/o-	contra-	-ar	dacryo-

<table>
<tr><td>B</td><td>I</td><td>N</td><td>G</td><td>O</td></tr>
<tr><td>choledoch/o-</td><td>capn/o-</td><td>coccyg/o-</td><td>caust/o-</td><td>episi/o-</td></tr>
<tr><td>conch/a-</td><td>abort/io</td><td>ana-</td><td>antr/o-</td><td>-clysis</td></tr>
<tr><td>faci/o-</td><td>-aria</td><td>FREE</td><td>an-</td><td>capill/o-</td></tr>
<tr><td>acoust/i-</td><td>dist/o-</td><td>dors/o-</td><td>brux-</td><td>-e</td></tr>
<tr><td>capit/o-</td><td>cerbr/o-</td><td>catheter/o-</td><td>-cele</td><td>eti/o-</td></tr>
</table>

<table>
<tr><td colspan="5" align="center"># B I N G O</td></tr>
<tr><td>clavicul/o-</td><td>ceno-</td><td>cebo-</td><td>Bacteri/o-</td><td>Benign/i-</td></tr>
<tr><td>eruct/o-</td><td>-or</td><td>cub/o-</td><td>-form</td><td>catarrh-</td></tr>
<tr><td>amnio-</td><td>cusp/i-</td><td>FREE</td><td>-flect</td><td>core/o-</td></tr>
<tr><td>acrom/i-</td><td>aponeur/o-</td><td>cirrh/o-</td><td>cleido-</td><td>cholangio-</td></tr>
<tr><td>DERMAT/O-</td><td>-cept-</td><td>eschar</td><td>cras/o-</td><td>-clas</td></tr>
</table>

B I N G O

B	I	N	G	O
Benign/i-	foc/o-	brady-	-centesis	decub/o-
clavicul/o-	ef-	cimex-	colon/o-	coagulo/o-
a-	abcess	FREE	-ary	fil-
fract/o-	DERMAT/O-	doch/o-	eschar	-ectomy
Bas/o-	-ellum	crani/o-	amnio-	deep

B	I	N	G	O
esthes/i-	chilo-	dia-	dacryo-	eso-
caud/o-	fil-	eccrine-	cistern/o-	a-
convolo-	Benign/i-	FREE	carp/o-	chordo- (cordo-)
cycl/o-	en-	cau-	ferro-	crypto-
cost/o-	-flect	ascar/i-	-cicatrix	access/o-

<table>
<tr><td>B</td><td>I</td><td>N</td><td>G</td><td>O</td></tr>
<tr><td>-ellum</td><td>-ar</td><td>-coccus</td><td>-borg</td><td>flagell/o-</td></tr>
<tr><td>fibrill/o-</td><td>dracuncul/o-</td><td>brady-</td><td>-crit</td><td>bol/o-</td></tr>
<tr><td>ferro-</td><td>carbun/o-</td><td>FREE</td><td>acrachn/</td><td>-us</td></tr>
<tr><td>duoden/o-</td><td>culd/o-</td><td>angi/o-</td><td>Bacteri/o-</td><td>amino-</td></tr>
<tr><td>anecto-</td><td>enamel</td><td>encephal/o-</td><td>cerbr/o-</td><td>scato-</td></tr>
</table>

B I N G O

B	I	N	G	O
cycl/o-	eruct/o-	centi-	comato-	culd/o-
antr/um-	-clas	candid/i-	asthma-	alb/o-
-enchyma	angin/o-	FREE	bronch/i-	keno-
aqua-	diaphoro-	-clast	-estasy	abdomin/o-
anecto-	alveol/i-	diplo-	e-	eczema

BINGO

B	I	N	G	O
-clast	fulv/o-	chiro-	abcess	coel-
-agon	Bil/i- (bil-)	cebo-	eu-	ana-
eczema	af-	FREE	fossa-	chilo-
gelat/o-	chondr/o-	diplo-	cili-	caput-
bulimo-	chlor/o-	auscult/o-	-emesis	eti/o-

B I N G O

B	I	N	G	O
diverticul/o-	abcess	-cytosis	angi/o-	amino-
dem/o-	cement/o-	bulba-	calcane/o-	corac/o-
actin/o-	-estasy	FREE	azygo-	entero-
anti-	emmetr/o-	e-	bronch/i-	dolich/o-
eczema	fibro-	dips/o-	capill/o-	fulgur/o-

<table>
<tr><td colspan="5" align="center"># B I N G O</td></tr>
<tr><td>brach/i-</td><td>chyle-</td><td>diplo-</td><td>delta</td><td>crenat/o-</td></tr>
<tr><td>dist/o-</td><td>acrachn/</td><td>contrecoup</td><td>cephalo-</td><td>carbun/o-</td></tr>
<tr><td>effus-</td><td>ab-</td><td>FREE</td><td>-creas</td><td>ante-</td></tr>
<tr><td>cyan/o-</td><td>axo-</td><td>fulgur/o-</td><td>blepharo-
(palpebro-)</td><td>gamet/o-</td></tr>
<tr><td>clubb/o-</td><td>-cid</td><td>enuresis-</td><td>caligi/o-</td><td>fet/o-</td></tr>
</table>

BINGO

B	I	N	G	O
capit/o-	carb/o-	dia-	centr/i-	edema-
chancr/o-	DEPRESS-	cau-	chyme-	arachino-
emphysema	ecto-	FREE	caus-	apo-
-e	aponeur/o-	flat/o-	-collis	gelatino-
-cece	condyl/o-	ab-	gamet/o-	-ellum

B I N G O

B	I	N	G	O
eti/o-	Bas/o-	anthrop/o-	ec-	gelat/o-
crust/-	dolich/o-	alb/o-	entero-	cune/i-
-clast	-e	FREE	acanth/o-	anthrac/o-
aponeur/o-	corac/o-	bula-	amblyo-	gangli/o-
dia-	-facient	deuter/o-	emac/i-	-crit

BINGO

B	I	N	G	O
chrom/o-	Bas/o-	fract/o-	adhes/io-	-algia
ex-	atelo-	erythermat/o-	anis/o-	centi-
cil/i-	chorea-	FREE	-deferens	carp/o-
-ellum	cyte-	acoust/i-	bula-	cyth-
aster/o-	gamet/o-	ec-	andr/o-	cal/o-

BINGO

B	I	N	G	O
dist/o-	ante-	comato-	-amine	emac/i-
chordo- (cordo-)	co-	facet	andr/o-	alopec/i-
anthr/o-	circum-	FREE	-cyesis	centr/i-
ethm/o-	enema	fila-	concuss/i-	arthr/o-
-or	avuls/i-	aut-	cement/o-	cholecyst/o-

B I N G O

B	I	N	G	O
fungi-	append/o-	cebo-	sterco-	dolich/o-
fili-	athero-	anxio-	cerbr/o-	formamen/o-
-amine	burs/o-	FREE	diplo-	a-
flex-	audi-	flagell/o-	chondr/o-	chlamyd/i-
chlor/o-	Balan/o-	cau-	alveol/i-	-crine

<table>
<tr><td>B</td><td>I</td><td>N</td><td>G</td><td>O</td></tr>
<tr><td>centr/i-</td><td>fimbri/o-</td><td>du/o-</td><td>cerbr/o-</td><td>auricul/o-</td></tr>
<tr><td>gelat/o-</td><td>-flect</td><td>extra-</td><td>-ectasis</td><td>alimento/o</td></tr>
<tr><td>ecchymo/-</td><td>keno-</td><td>FREE</td><td>Benign/i-</td><td>axo-</td></tr>
<tr><td>auto-</td><td>acrom/i-</td><td>bula-</td><td>coccyg/o-</td><td>corp/o-</td></tr>
<tr><td>dextr/o-</td><td>capit/o-</td><td>acu-</td><td>clon/o-</td><td>sterco-</td></tr>
</table>

B	I	N	G	O
adip/o-	aster/o-	cerv/i-	cement/o-	antr/o-
cirrh/o-	delta	-ition	cyte-	debride-
ef-	-ory	FREE	calcane/o-	dy/o-
cystido-	asthma-	fistul/o-	centro-	arteri/o-
chiasma	Bas/io-	fontan/o-	Bacill/o	cycl/o-

BINGO

B	I	N	G	O
co-	fec/o-	comato-	colob/o-	col/o-
DERM/O-	chiro-	ante-	centr/i-	catarrh-
duct/o-	calx-	FREE	an/o-	anecto-
emac/i-	bula-	duoden/o-	-atresia	asco-
desmo-	gelatino-	-al	cyst/o-	clubb/o-

<table>
<tr><td>B</td><td>I</td><td>N</td><td>G</td><td>O</td></tr>
<tr><td>auscult/o-</td><td>ankyl/o-</td><td>cornu-</td><td>ethm/o-</td><td>ante-</td></tr>
<tr><td>ana-</td><td>-amine</td><td>eosin/o-</td><td>-artresia</td><td>corp/o-</td></tr>
<tr><td>acu-</td><td>alb/o-</td><td>FREE</td><td>cryo-</td><td>abort/io</td></tr>
<tr><td>debride-</td><td>fistul/o-</td><td>gelat/o-</td><td>fulv/o-</td><td>-er</td></tr>
<tr><td>anil/i-</td><td>flat/o-</td><td>chalaz/io-</td><td>centr/i-</td><td>gangren/o-</td></tr>
</table>

BINGO

B	I	N	G	O
ab-	ecchymo/-	auto-	anter/o-	-coccus
carp/o-	erthr/o-	electr/o-	febr/o-	furun/o-
erythermat/o-	femor/o-	FREE	dacryo-	cori/o-
clon/o-	-ar	encephal/o-	anthrop/o-	enema
-dynia	-amine	articul/o-	ferro-	ankyl/o-

B	I	N	G	O	
B	I	N	G	O	without or lack of
B	I	N	G	O	away (away from)
B	I	N	G	O	belly
B	I	N	G	O	capable of
B	I	N	G	O	to miscarry or miscarrying (natural or induced)
B	I	N	G	O	to tear away from
B	I	N	G	O	a going away
B	I	N	G	O	refers to or pertains to
B	I	N	G	O	refers to or pertains to
B	I	N	G	O	refers to or pertains to
B	I	N	G	O	thorny (skin growth)
B	I	N	G	O	supplemental
B	I	N	G	O	vinegar cup or hip joint (for femur)
B	I	N	G	O	pointed
B	I	N	G	O	hearing
B	I	N	G	O	extremities, height and pointed
B	I	N	G	O	extremities, height and pointed
B	I	N	G	O	sun, ray, radium
B	I	N	G	O	sharp
B	I	N	G	O	sharp
B	I	N	G	O	near or beside
B	I	N	G	O	gland
B	I	N	G	O	to stick (together)
B	I	N	G	O	fat
B	I	N	G	O	air or gas
B	I	N	G	O	toward
B	I	N	G	O	relates to or pertains to
B	I	N	G	O	to clump
B	I	N	G	O	inducing or leading
B	I	N	G	O	walls
B	I	N	G	O	pain
B	I	N	G	O	refers to
B	I	N	G	O	white
B	I	N	G	O	egg white
B	I	N	G	O	pain
B	I	N	G	O	pain
B	I	N	G	O	to nourish
B	I	N	G	O	fox mange or baldness
B	I	N	G	O	cavity
B	I	N	G	O	both
B	I	N	G	O	dull
B	I	N	G	O	to walk
B	I	N	G	O	nitrogen compound
B	I	N	G	O	organic compound
B	I	N	G	O	forgetful

B	I	N	G	O	
B	I	N	G	O	lambs caul 'small cap'
B	I	N	G	O	both
B	I	N	G	O	starch
B	I	N	G	O	lack of or without
B	I	N	G	O	ring
B	I	N	G	O	apart or up
B	I	N	G	O	elbow
B	I	N	G	O	man or male
B	I	N	G	O	without expansion or dilation
B	I	N	G	O	vessel
B	I	N	G	O	to choke
B	I	N	G	O	old women
B	I	N	G	O	unequal
B	I	N	G	O	fuse or bind
B	I	N	G	O	abnormal
B	I	N	G	O	before
B	I	N	G	O	before or foremost (in front)
B	I	N	G	O	coal or carbuncle
B	I	N	G	O	coal or carbuncle
B	I	N	G	O	human
B	I	N	G	O	against
B	I	N	G	O	cavity
B	I	N	G	O	cavity or cavern
B	I	N	G	O	dilation or ballooning
B	I	N	G	O	restlessness, uneasy, apprehensive
B	I	N	G	O	to remove or separate
B	I	N	G	O	above or upon
B	I	N	G	O	upon tendon (sheet or sheath around tendon)
B	I	N	G	O	appendage
B	I	N	G	O	water
B	I	N	G	O	refers to
B	I	N	G	O	without or lack of
B	I	N	G	O	spider
B	I	N	G	O	spider
B	I	N	G	O	first
B	I	N	G	O	first
B	I	N	G	O	air
B	I	N	G	O	artery
B	I	N	G	O	joint
B	I	N	G	O	jointed
B	I	N	G	O	refers to
B	I	N	G	O	unquenchable
B	I	N	G	O	worm
B	I	N	G	O	bag
B	I	N	G	O	enzyme

B	I	N	G	O	
B	I	N	G	O	to sprinkle
B	I	N	G	O	star
B	I	N	G	O	weakness
B	I	N	G	O	panting
B	I	N	G	O	refers to or action
B	I	N	G	O	incomplete, without end, imperfect (ending)
B	I	N	G	O	porridge or yellow fat
B	I	N	G	O	process of or procedure of
B	I	N	G	O	process of or procedure of
B	I	N	G	O	vapor or steam
B	I	N	G	O	closure
B	I	N	G	O	chamber
B	I	N	G	O	wearing out
B	I	N	G	O	hearing
B	I	N	G	O	ear
B	I	N	G	O	ear
B	I	N	G	O	to listen
B	I	N	G	O	self
B	I	N	G	O	self
B	I	N	G	O	to tear
B	I	N	G	O	armpit or central
B	I	N	G	O	axle or axis
B	I	N	G	O	axle or axis
B	I	N	G	O	urea nitrogen
B	I	N	G	O	single
B	I	N	G	O	ROD-LIKE
B	I	N	G	O	ROD
B	I	N	G	O	PENIS (GLANS PENIS)
B	I	N	G	O	WEIGHT
B	I	N	G	O	HEAVY
B	I	N	G	O	basic
B	I	N	G	O	at a base
B	I	N	G	O	good or normal
B	I	N	G	O	kind
B	I	N	G	O	weakness
B	I	N	G	O	two
B	I	N	G	O	bile or gall
B	I	N	G	O	two
B	I	N	G	O	life
B	I	N	G	O	beginning or young
B	I	N	G	O	blister
B	I	N	G	O	mucus
B	I	N	G	O	eyelid
B	I	N	G	O	lump or ball
B	I	N	G	O	orgasm

B	I	N	G	O	
B	I	N	G	O	arm
B	I	N	G	O	short
B	I	N	G	O	slow
B	I	N	G	O	short
B	I	N	G	O	windpipe or tracea-like
B	I	N	G	O	grinding
B	I	N	G	O	cheek
B	I	N	G	O	bister or vesicle
B	I	N	G	O	blister or vesicle
B	I	N	G	O	hunger
B	I	N	G	O	sac, wine-sac, or pouch
B	I	N	G	O	diseased or bad
B	I	N	G	O	heat, heated or hot
B	I	N	G	O	heel
B	I	N	G	O	calcium
B	I	N	G	O	pebbles or granules (of calcium mineral)
B	I	N	G	O	dim vision
B	I	N	G	O	cups
B	I	N	G	O	cups
B	I	N	G	O	hardened skin
B	I	N	G	O	heel or lime
B	I	N	G	O	glowing white
B	I	N	G	O	corner of eye
B	I	N	G	O	hair-like
B	I	N	G	O	head
B	I	N	G	O	carbon dioxide
B	I	N	G	O	little box
B	I	N	G	O	head
B	I	N	G	O	carbon atoms, coal, or charcoal
B	I	N	G	O	glowing ember
B	I	N	G	O	glowing ember
B	I	N	G	O	crab-like
B	I	N	G	O	heart
B	I	N	G	O	wrist
B	I	N	G	O	breakdown or down
B	I	N	G	O	waterfall or cloudiness
B	I	N	G	O	to flow down
B	I	N	G	O	to let down into
B	I	N	G	O	tall or toward tall
B	I	N	G	O	burn or heat
B	I	N	G	O	burn or heat
B	I	N	G	O	burn or heat
B	I	N	G	O	hollow
B	I	N	G	O	meal or food
B	I	N	G	O	blind pouch

B	I	N	G	O	
B	I	N	G	O	navel
B	I	N	G	O	swelling or tumor
B	I	N	G	O	abdomen or belly
B	I	N	G	O	chambers
B	I	N	G	O	hard
B	I	N	G	O	empty or common
B	I	N	G	O	empty or common
B	I	N	G	O	surgical puncture to drain fluid
B	I	N	G	O	one-hundredth apart
B	I	N	G	O	center
B	I	N	G	O	center
B	I	N	G	O	head
B	I	N	G	O	receiver
B	I	N	G	O	brain
B	I	N	G	O	wax
B	I	N	G	O	neck
B	I	N	G	O	relaxation
B	I	N	G	O	hailstone (eyelid sebaceous cyst)
B	I	N	G	O	ulcer (sore)
B	I	N	G	O	lip
B	I	N	G	O	lip
B	I	N	G	O	a crossing
B	I	N	G	O	hand
B	I	N	G	O	to cloak or cover
B	I	N	G	O	green
B	I	N	G	O	bile duct
B	I	N	G	O	bile or gall (ingredient of)
B	I	N	G	O	gallbladder
B	I	N	G	O	gallbladder duct (canal)
B	I	N	G	O	billary acute diarrhea
B	I	N	G	O	cartilage
B	I	N	G	O	cord
B	I	N	G	O	dancing (shaking)
B	I	N	G	O	colored
B	I	N	G	O	juice
B	I	N	G	O	juice
B	I	N	G	O	scar
B	I	N	G	O	to kill
B	I	N	G	O	eyelash-like
B	I	N	G	O	eyelash or eyelash like
B	I	N	G	O	bug
B	I	N	G	O	movement filming
B	I	N	G	O	around
B	I	N	G	O	yellow-oranged (jaundiced)
B	I	N	G	O	cut or to cut

B	I	N	G	O	
B	I	N	G	O	cavity
B	I	N	G	O	relaxation
B	I	N	G	O	breakdown
B	I	N	G	O	breakdown
B	I	N	G	O	collar bone (little key shape)
B	I	N	G	O	hook, clavicle or collar bone
B	I	N	G	O	bent
B	I	N	G	O	turmoil
B	I	N	G	O	rounding
B	I	N	G	O	irrigation or injection
B	I	N	G	O	two
B	I	N	G	O	clotting or clot
B	I	N	G	O	berry
B	I	N	G	O	tailbone
B	I	N	G	O	snail-like
B	I	N	G	O	hollow belly (cavity)
B	I	N	G	O	to come together (sexual union; inter/course "between/a flowing")
B	I	N	G	O	colon big or large intestine
B	I	N	G	O	colon big or large intestine
B	I	N	G	O	glue
B	I	N	G	O	twisted
B	I	N	G	O	to mutilate
B	I	N	G	O	vagina
B	I	N	G	O	together
B	I	N	G	O	deep sleep
B	I	N	G	O	together
B	I	N	G	O	shell
B	I	N	G	O	violent shaking
B	I	N	G	O	knuckle (nob)
B	I	N	G	O	dust
B	I	N	G	O	cone shaped
B	I	N	G	O	together joined (united)
B	I	N	G	O	contained
B	I	N	G	O	against
B	I	N	G	O	counter blow
B	I	N	G	O	bruise
B	I	N	G	O	to roll together
B	I	N	G	O	crows beak (shape)
B	I	N	G	O	vocal chords cord
B	I	N	G	O	pupil or iris (rainbow)
B	I	N	G	O	skin
B	I	N	G	O	cornea or horn (shape)
B	I	N	G	O	horn or horny
B	I	N	G	O	crowning
B	I	N	G	O	crowning frontal body cut

B	I	N	G	O	
B	I	N	G	O	body
B	I	N	G	O	bark, outer bark, rind, or cortex
B	I	N	G	O	rib
B	I	N	G	O	hip, hip joint, (pelvis and femur)
B	I	N	G	O	hip, hip joint, (pelvis and femur)
B	I	N	G	O	skull
B	I	N	G	O	mixture
B	I	N	G	O	fleshy or flesh
B	I	N	G	O	notched
B	I	N	G	O	ring
B	I	N	G	O	secrete
B	I	N	G	O	secrete
B	I	N	G	O	separate
B	I	N	G	O	cross or cross-like
B	I	N	G	O	leg thigh or femur
B	I	N	G	O	leg thigh or femur
B	I	N	G	O	scab or outer coat
B	I	N	G	O	cold
B	I	N	G	O	secret
B	I	N	G	O	cube or cube shaped
B	I	N	G	O	elbow
B	I	N	G	O	blind pouch
B	I	N	G	O	little
B	I	N	G	O	wedge
B	I	N	G	O	scooping or scraping
B	I	N	G	O	hearing
B	I	N	G	O	pointed
B	I	N	G	O	skin
B	I	N	G	O	skin
B	I	N	G	O	blue
B	I	N	G	O	circle
B	I	N	G	O	pregnancy
B	I	N	G	O	bladder or sac
B	I	N	G	O	bladder or sac
B	I	N	G	O	bladder or sac
B	I	N	G	O	bladder or sac
B	I	N	G	O	cell or chamber
B	I	N	G	O	cell or chamber
B	I	N	G	O	cell or chamber
B	I	N	G	O	increase (in number)
B	I	N	G	O	tear
B	I	N	G	O	digits (fingers and toes)
B	I	N	G	O	away
B	I	N	G	O	removal
B	I	N	G	O	one/tenth (1/10)

B	I	N	G	O	
B	I	N	G	O	one/tenth (1/10)
B	I	N	G	O	to lie down
B	I	N	G	O	most inward
B	I	N	G	O	ten
B	I	N	G	O	fan shaped or triangular
B	I	N	G	O	people
B	I	N	G	O	half
B	I	N	G	O	tree-shaped
B	I	N	G	O	TOOTH OR TEETH
B	I	N	G	O	TOOTH OR TEETH
B	I	N	G	O	LOWER
B	I	N	G	O	SKIN
B	I	N	G	O	SKIN
B	I	N	G	O	BINDING, TO BAND OR A BAND
B	I	N	G	O	ligament (also tendon)
B	I	N	G	O	second or secondary
B	I	N	G	O	rght
B	I	N	G	O	two
B	I	N	G	O	across, through, total or complete, or between
B	I	N	G	O	excessive sweating
B	I	N	G	O	testis or teste
B	I	N	G	O	to separate or apart
B	I	N	G	O	to separate or apart
B	I	N	G	O	finger or toe
B	I	N	G	O	double or two
B	I	N	G	O	thirst or thirsty
B	I	N	G	O	membrane
B	I	N	G	O	away from or reversed
B	I	N	G	O	farther from
B	I	N	G	O	outpouching
B	I	N	G	O	duct or canal
B	I	N	G	O	to teach or teacher
B	I	N	G	O	pain
B	I	N	G	O	long, seperation, dislocation
B	I	N	G	O	back
B	I	N	G	O	a giving
B	I	N	G	O	what is given
B	I	N	G	O	little dragon (worm)
B	I	N	G	O	running
B	I	N	G	O	two
B	I	N	G	O	to draw or to lead (motion) away
B	I	N	G	O	twelve
B	I	N	G	O	hard
B	I	N	G	O	small
B	I	N	G	O	two or a pair

B	I	N	G	O	
B	I	N	G	O	work or strength
B	I	N	G	O	pain
B	I	N	G	O	diffucult, faulty or painful
B	I	N	G	O	instrument
B	I	N	G	O	out or remove
B	I	N	G	O	refers to
B	I	N	G	O	outside, outward, outer or out
B	I	N	G	O	outside, outward, outer or out
B	I	N	G	O	outside, outward, outer or out
B	I	N	G	O	juice out
B	I	N	G	O	secreting or to secrete
B	I	N	G	O	prickly, spiny or notched
B	I	N	G	O	sound
B	I	N	G	O	dilation
B	I	N	G	O	dilation
B	I	N	G	O	excisio or removal
B	I	N	G	O	to boil out
B	I	N	G	O	swelling
B	I	N	G	O	away or out
B	I	N	G	O	away or out
B	I	N	G	O	away or out
B	I	N	G	O	electrical
B	I	N	G	O	lesser or smaller
B	I	N	G	O	in
B	I	N	G	O	to grow thin
B	I	N	G	O	early
B	I	N	G	O	vomit
B	I	N	G	O	blood
B	I	N	G	O	normal or correct
B	I	N	G	O	puffed up
B	I	N	G	O	in
B	I	N	G	O	hard
B	I	N	G	O	within head brain
B	I	N	G	O	anything poured in (essential organ part)
B	I	N	G	O	within or inside
B	I	N	G	O	injection
B	I	N	G	O	intestine (usually refers to small intestine)
B	I	N	G	O	to void (expel) urine
B	I	N	G	O	rose red (color)
B	I	N	G	O	upon
B	I	N	G	O	pubic region
B	I	N	G	O	one who
B	I	N	G	O	one who
B	I	N	G	O	work or labor
B	I	N	G	O	belching

B	I	N	G	O	
B	I	N	G	O	red or flushed
B	I	N	G	O	red
B	I	N	G	O	scab
B	I	N	G	O	toward
B	I	N	G	O	feeling (physical)
B	I	N	G	O	female
B	I	N	G	O	sieve
B	I	N	G	O	cause
B	I	N	G	O	cause
B	I	N	G	O	good or normal
B	I	N	G	O	out, outside, outward
B	I	N	G	O	out, outside, outward
B	I	N	G	O	out, outside, outward
B	I	N	G	O	face
B	I	N	G	O	face
B	I	N	G	O	face
B	I	N	G	O	making
B	I	N	G	O	band
B	I	N	G	O	fever
B	I	N	G	O	stool, fecal matter, or dung
B	I	N	G	O	stool, fecal matter, or dung
B	I	N	G	O	srool, fecal matter or dung
B	I	N	G	O	thigh
B	I	N	G	O	window
B	I	N	G	O	to carry
B	I	N	G	O	iron
B	I	N	G	O	young
B	I	N	G	O	to quiver
B	I	N	G	O	fiber-like
B	I	N	G	O	fiber
B	I	N	G	O	to clasp
B	I	N	G	O	thread
B	I	N	G	O	thread
B	I	N	G	O	thread
B	I	N	G	O	thread
B	I	N	G	O	fingers
B	I	N	G	O	to split or splitting
B	I	N	G	O	pipe or pipe-stem
B	I	N	G	O	soft
B	I	N	G	O	whip
B	I	N	G	O	to blow
B	I	N	G	O	to bend
B	I	N	G	O	to bend
B	I	N	G	O	flowing
B	I	N	G	O	to flow

B	I	N	G	O	
B	I	N	G	O	center or hearth
B	I	N	G	O	little fountain
B	I	N	G	O	opening
B	I	N	G	O	before
B	I	N	G	O	shaped shape or form
B	I	N	G	O	furrow or shallow depression
B	I	N	G	O	to break
B	I	N	G	O	forehead or before
B	I	N	G	O	to flee
B	I	N	G	O	to lighten (with sparks burning tissue)
B	I	N	G	O	brown
B	I	N	G	O	base or lage part (organ body)
B	I	N	G	O	mushroom
B	I	N	G	O	branch or fork
B	I	N	G	O	boil
B	I	N	G	O	milk
B	I	N	G	O	to marry, unite, or sexual union
B	I	N	G	O	to marry, unite, or sexual union
B	I	N	G	O	knot swelling or collection knot
B	I	N	G	O	eating sore
B	I	N	G	O	stomach
B	I	N	G	O	freeze or congeal
B	I	N	G	O	freeze or congeal

PREFIXES & SUFFIXES -

Medical Terminology Activity

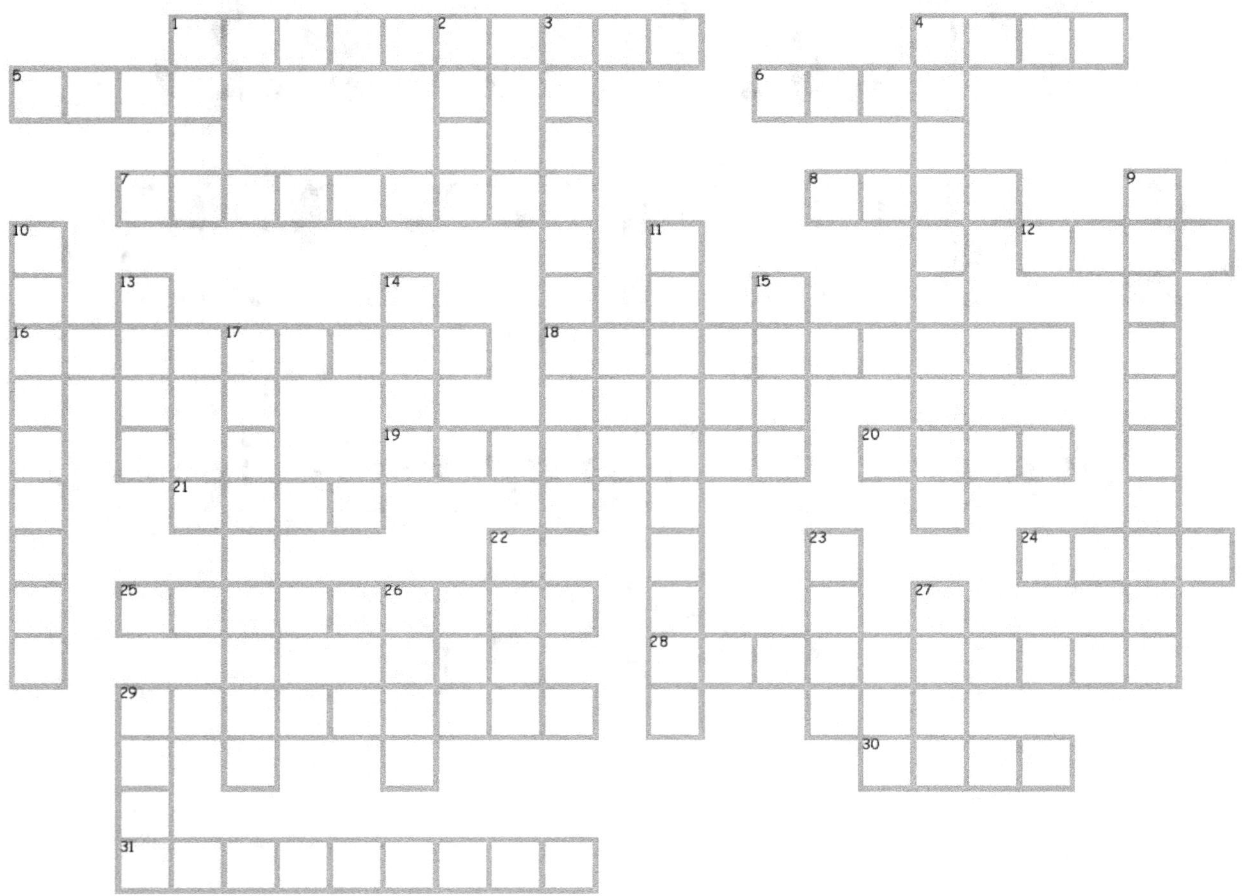

Across

1 gallbladder duct (canal)
4 pointed
5 both
6 to split or splitting
7 to separate or apart
8 to bend
12 breakdown
16 bile duct
18 together joined (united)
19 egg white
20 to flow
21 air or gas
24 sharp
25 vinegar cup or hip joint (for femur)
28 gallbladder
29 to nourish
30 before
31 puffed up

Down

1 eyelash-like
2 what is given
3 counter blow
4 to sprinkle
9 glowing ember
10 within head brain
11 contained
13 center or hearth
14 thread
15 self
17 to remove or separate
22 white
23 thread
26 good or normal
27 extremities, height and pointed
29 capable of

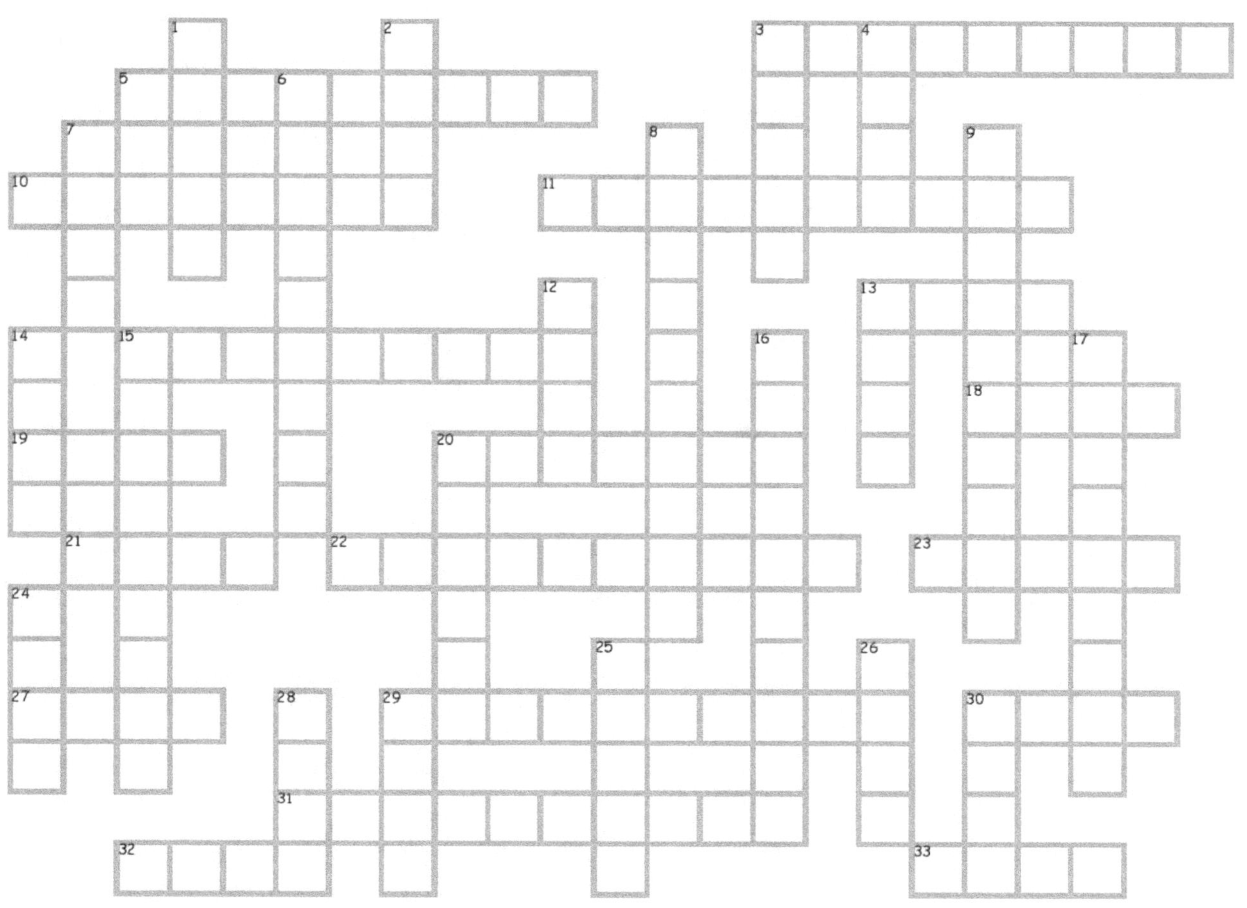

Across

3 within head brain
5 to separate or apart
10 ROD
11 gallbladder duct (canal)
13 blister or vesicle
15 to nourish
18 heat, heated or hot
19 sound
20 billary acute diarrhea
21 grinding
22 counter blow
23 chamber
27 secrete
29 glowing ember
30 swelling or tumor
31 together joined (united)
32 blind pouch
33 burn or heat

Down

1 farther from
2 cold
3 away or out
4 meal or food
6 opening
7 heel or lime
8 contained
9 gallbladder
12 lump or ball
13 WEIGHT
14 hollow belly (cavity)
15 to remove or separate
16 little dragon (worm)
17 collar bone (little key shape)
20 shell
24 navel
25 to draw or to lead (motion) away
26 orgasm
28 diseased or bad
29 empty or common
30 breakdown or down

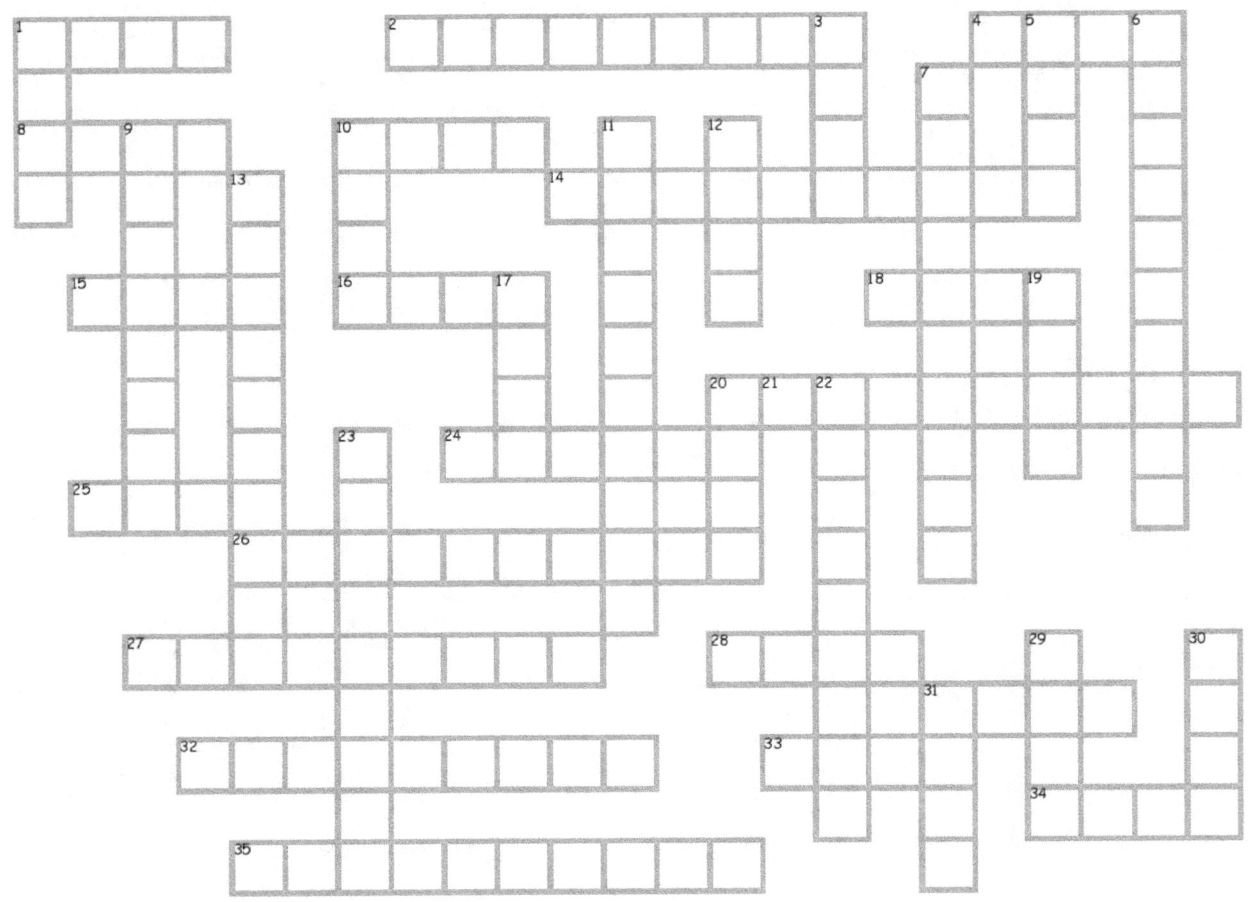

Across

1 heat, heated or hot
2 puffed up
4 breakdown or down
8 breakdown
10 against
14 contained
15 self
16 pain
18 blister or vesicle
21 vinegar cup or hip joint (for femur)
24 berry
25 lump or ball
26 glowing ember
27 bile duct
28 diseased or bad
31 WEIGHT
32 within head brain
33 white
34 hearing
35 gallbladder

Down

1 blind pouch
3 walls
5 before
6 to sprinkle
7 together joined (united)
9 to tear away from
10 water
11 counter blow
12 vapor or steam
13 gallbladder duct (canal)
17 air or gas
19 both
20 bag
22 collar bone (little key shape)
23 opening
29 air
30 ear
31 orgasm

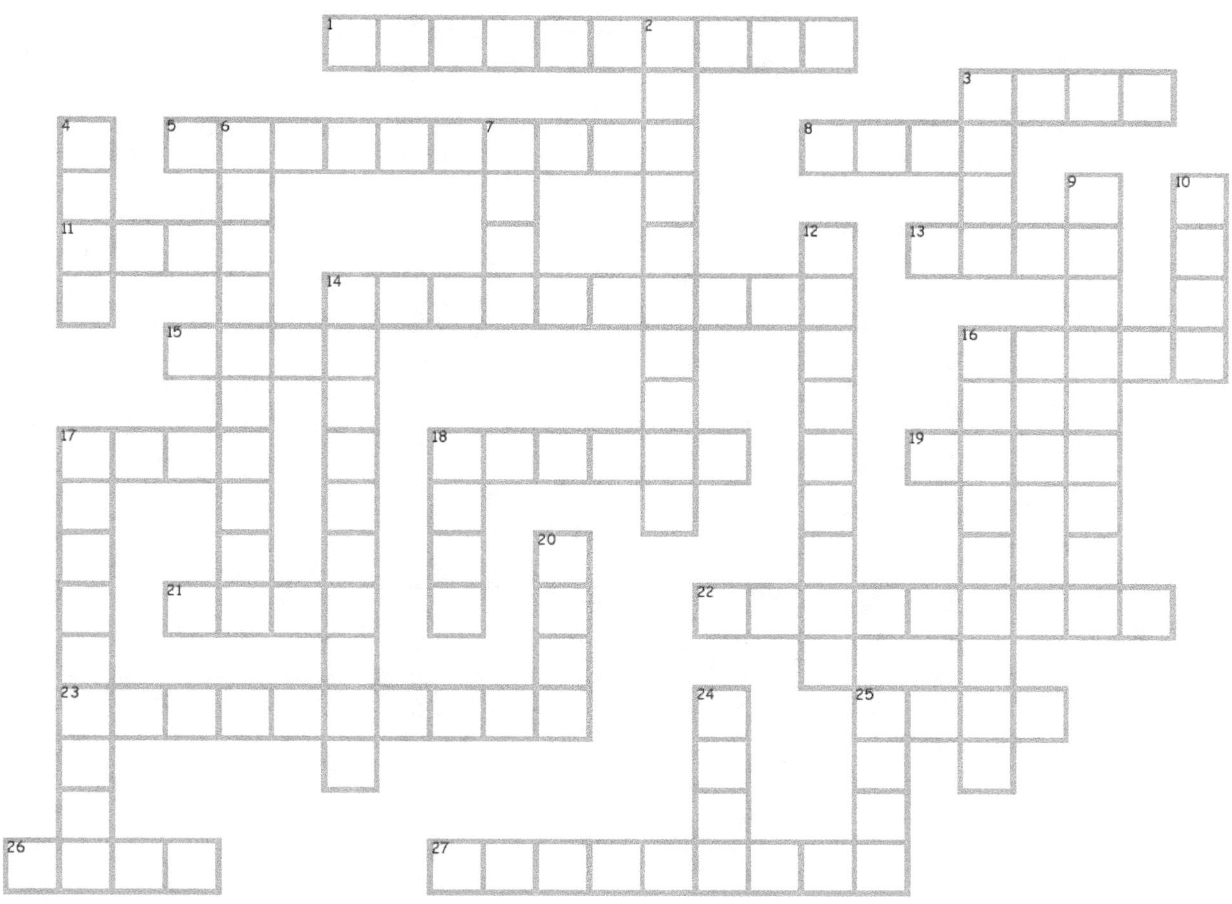

Across

1. little dragon (worm)
3. bladder or sac
5. glowing ember
8. wax
11. most inward
13. people
14. counter blow
15. cold
16. bug
17. eyelash-like
18. head
19. shaped shape or form
21. what is given
22. to nourish
23. together joined (united)
25. secrete
26. hip, hip joint, (pelvis and femur)
27. within head brain

Down

2. gallbladder
3. little
4. within or inside
6. to sprinkle
7. separate
9. opening
10. to bend
12. to remove or separate
14. contained
16. bile duct
17. collar bone (little key shape)
18. vocal chords cord
20. hip, hip joint, (pelvis and femur)
24. cell or chamber
25. cube or cube shaped

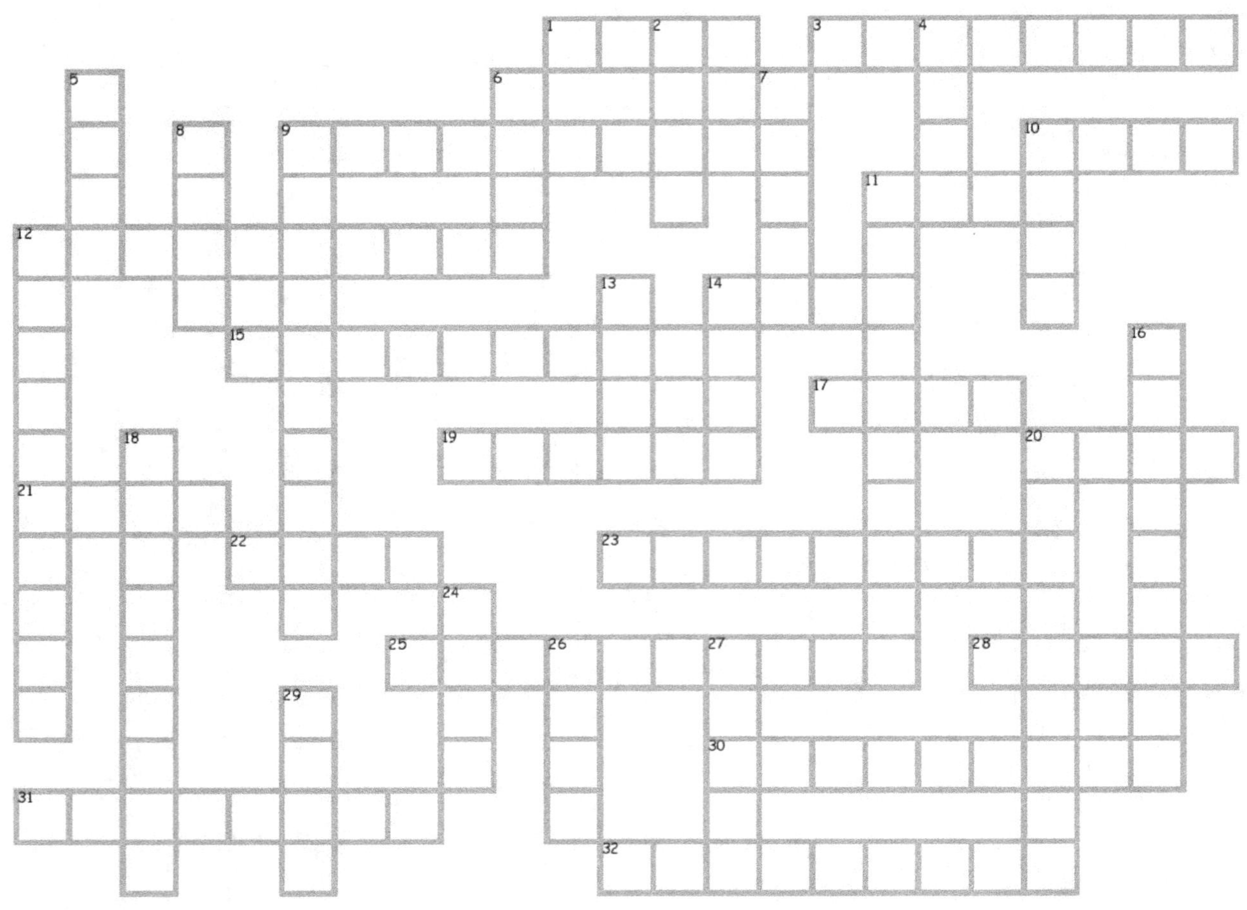

Across

1 navel
3 egg white
9 gallbladder duct (canal)
10 grinding
11 diseased or bad
12 contained
14 WEIGHT
15 little dragon (worm)
17 weakness
19 sun, ray, radium
20 breakdown or down
21 heat, heated or hot
22 ear
23 puffed up
25 glowing ember
28 bug
30 vinegar cup or hip joint (for femur)
31 upon tendon (sheet or sheath around tendon)
32 bile duct

Down

2 blind pouch
4 blister or vesicle
5 axle or axis
6 good or normal
7 furrow or shallow depression
8 self
9 counter blow
10 orgasm
11 gallbladder
12 together joined (united)
13 hearing
14 lump or ball
16 to let down into
18 to nourish
20 collar bone (little key shape)
24 HEAVY
26 basic
27 mixture
29 burn or heat

PREFIXES & SUFFIXES Word Search Puzzle

```
Q T O H R O D E T A E H T A E H W K B W H R R J Q Z F E C O T A B Q B
R O R G A S M S G O A T K D K A A L Q O A E R T H R O L Q H L Y C V J
A I Q O B B U L C Y P G Z V L R A N T T O T O L U S P A C G M W H F I
E D N H G P F O Z L O L S U F D F Z N S K M E W O L B R E T N U O E X
T A N I G A V F R E B I D M M D U W P F F U R T F K S G N I R A E H
O Y U I N Q J J R G M F Y I E A A L N T R E Z N E V B O I C T G B D X P
T D Q I I C Y B C A P W R E F L A G R F G S W R R R R N T C O R N E A
R X N Q K W O D P O R O M M L O L D U E T W W R O H A I R Q I A C B N
I J Y A S D A N T H R A C O P C C F J R C T E G N T E C C D M N P G T
H O A L H W M B T S A R O U N D A O O E O T Y T C N R F Y R S L D G I
R J G A A C R Y A U D J G Z I I L L K B S T V V H A O M F E A R X C
M Y H Y O C O C I H S W X I A M L E D I R B E D I U A G C U S C V Z C
Z D H X Z C F Z Y G E I Y S P N O V L F B C B Q E L C R I C S I M Y D U
H A O B M A B O V M A N E C T O Z B Z V P O C G H L Q E S I E Y S D U
T O H T N A C A R E B M A H C R O L L E C E S C O I L G N A G E S U
```

☐ANTI-
☐REFERS TO
☐HARD
☐FEC/O-
☐ERTHR/O-
☐FIBER
☐AZYGO-
☐CALYX-
☐BLISTER
☐CIRCLE
☐ANTHR/O-
☐CARCIN/O-
☐ALGES/I-
☐DEBRIDE-
☐GANGLI/O-
☐AMBLYO-
☐-FORM

☐CORNE/O-
☐SMALL
☐BLADDER OR SAC
☐CLUBB/O-
☐HAND
☐AROUND
☐TO TEAR
☐COX/O-
☐WATER
☐CHLAMYD/I-
☐CALL/O-
☐ANTHRAC/O-
☐AER/O-
☐EFFUS-
☐ANECTO-
☐COUNTER BLOW

☐ACANTH/O-
☐BRONCH/I-
☐SKIN
☐VAGINA
☐ESTR/O-
☐CAPSULO-
☐HEAT, HEATED OR HOT
☐FULGUR/O-
☐ORGASM
☐PAIN
☐FOC/O-
☐CELL OR CHAMBER
☐-CYESIS
☐CONTUS/I-
☐HEARING
☐CLEIDO-

PREFIXES & SUFFIXES Word Search Puzzle

```
I J W S U Z W E A K N E S S A K I N D J C M I W M T A Q R F G S B K W
O Q D R O C S D R O H C L A C O V S D E D I M R I T M L R Y Y Y F R M
R H O R O H P A I D B V H D R J Z U M R D P R J L T Y S E G X L H E Y
U P Q F M O B L X R R O G U O A R P A E E W I C K N L O W Y E E H B Z
E E L E C T R O R B L E C N M N D W X U E C V U U E O L O S Z C C M A
N A N X N X B A O L O N D O I K O P E O P L E R R M H U L P A C Z E P
O V K C P E K T O B N C W I N T N I O J S U Q W Y U V C N M W R D G A
P O S U L A S W W Q O H I W P D N K F Z L A T H E R O I O D N I G N R
A Z T T U R I A J F R Y R H W S Y A Q L E Z Z S B T W T I E Q N F I T
A E A L E Y H N T Z O M G L A N D L P M E U T Z Z S S R T C I E Y W O
L I T F U L L A M S C A U C H Y L E O F P Y S A E N U E I D S H G O R
L X E X D C G N U O Y R O G N I N N I G E B Z V Y I K V N I A A E L U
U R E L C I S E V R O R E T I S I L C A R C I N O U B I Z R F W F G P
D K P A C I R U D N N T Z F R R O S E R E D C O L O R D D O R E T N E
H N K T P A F I A C C O N J U C T I V O W U G Z S G R E H T E G O T M
```

- ☐ CONDYL/O-
- ☐ CONJUCTIV/O-
- ☐ AUSCULT/O-
- ☐ BLISTER OR VESICLE
- ☐ TOWARD
- ☐ SPIDER
- ☐ VOCAL CHORDS CORD
- ☐ ATHERO-
- ☐ PAIN
- ☐ CHYLE-
- ☐ GLOWING EMBER
- ☐ DIAPHORO-
- ☐ AMYLO-
- ☐ KIND
- ☐ CORON/O-
- ☐ HARD
- ☐ ECCRINE-
- ☐ PEOPLE
- ☐ -ENCHYMA
- ☐ ELECTR/O-
- ☐ SMALL
- ☐ DEEP SLEEP
- ☐ REFERS TO
- ☐ DULL
- ☐ WEAKNESS
- ☐ CIRCUM-
- ☐ UNEASY
- ☐ APART OR UP
- ☐ PANTING
- ☐ HOLLOW
- ☐ APONEUR/O-
- ☐ ENTERO-
- ☐ TOGETHER
- ☐ -ITION
- ☐ ACROM/I-
- ☐ LOWER
- ☐ LITTLE BOX
- ☐ ROSE RED (COLOR)
- ☐ BEGINNING OR YOUNG
- ☐ STOMACH
- ☐ INSTRUMENT
- ☐ GRINDING
- ☐ DIVERTICUL/O-
- ☐ GLAND
- ☐ MILK
- ☐ SELF
- ☐ FASC/I-
- ☐ CARCIN/O-
- ☐ JOINT

PREFIXES & SUFFIXES Word Search Puzzle

T D E N I A T N O C J A C O R N U S O G Y C C O C C M O T S Y C N E K
A O D R O C O D R O H C U C H R O M O O O O A R O F A N T T I P X E D Q
A N N O G P T F A I S E R T R A L U U W R R V R C L A N X O Y R X O H Z Z A
T L N T B U X I R T A C I C I T U H V N R C D F E I O E Y A E S H S Z Z
H I L O H C A W A Y O R O U T C T M E Q O C I R N N R Y H M E R S J R A
R M I D I O R M O X R P Z O F O U R P T F Z O M X E M S Z D O S J J I N
A L P G I T R C C M K G X A P A O L I O S S U A L H A H O N Q T V E A N
C J W P L R S T P T S Y C O E F K C O T R N W J F T L S O C U X D A S E
O I S Y E O U W E P A E R Y E X I I A E I B I A G S E L M O Y X X S Q I
D U H F T T I S O E T H D Y T L T E C C N U A A F A O H R T E T I E I X
C V I D N U B X S Z T L E H I A L L B E C O Y L G C W O J G T S E Q P H
P W U E L C C H R N C H W Q X C U T K C F U Z Z L A Y C I M E D T P P H
U I B N O I T C A R O O T S R E F E R I M O R C A A F F Y D A K B P H O
E X C E S S I V E S W E A T I N G C M U K U O B W F E B R O F K P I W
B L E N N O B C I R C L E A N C O N E J G O C A D N I A P B C Q P Y W

- ☐ TOOTH OR TEETH
- ☐ FACET
- ☐ AURICUL/O-
- ☐ CHROM/O-
- ☐ LUMP OR BALL
- ☐ -DESIS
- ☐ ULCER (SORE)
- ☐ COLON/O-
- ☐ AWAY OR OUT
- ☐ CIRCLE
- ☐ ANTHROP/O-
- ☐ CILI-
- ☐ BOIL
- ☐ BRUCCA-
- ☐ CONTAINED
- ☐ -ARTRESIA
- ☐ AWAY OR OUT
- ☐ CYTE-
- ☐ PAIN
- ☐ CALX-
- ☐ CUSP/I-
- ☐ EXCESSIVE SWEATING
- ☐ RING
- ☐ DESMO-
- ☐ PAIN
- ☐ DOS/E- (DOSE)
- ☐ CUT OR TO CUT
- ☐ JUICE
- ☐ FEBR/O-
- ☐ DEMI-
- ☐ CYST/O-
- ☐ CORNU-
- ☐ REFERS TO OR ACTION
- ☐ MAN OR MALE
- ☐ CORNER OF EYE
- ☐ SHARP
- ☐ ACROM/I-
- ☐ ATTRIT/I-
- ☐ -ASTHENIA
- ☐ BENT
- ☐ COCCYG/O-
- ☐ CHORDO- (CORDO-)
- ☐ ANTHRAC/O-
- ☐ AGAINST
- ☐ BLENNO-
- ☐ CARDI/O-
- ☐ -CICATRIX
- ☐ ANCONE-

PREFIXES & SUFFIXES Word Search Puzzle

```
C R O U F M O C L A C C I S A B O K T A E H R O N R U B U W U Q M L Q
O S Y F H O H U F Y V Z L D G P U S D S T J I 0 T P K X A M U B I I Z
N W T G E O R S P A C L V E N M U H D Y S D G 1 O G R W N D G F X T U
I Y I L R C A M N O A Z A E U U L X V K A S O 1 L N T A P S O Q T T F
O U V A A G J T R J G I C A S M C V D W L B H C R J O H S O G T U L D
X T A G R J U U J U S C O L X O O M I P B E A T R J O H T S G R E C H
J K C O Z X X K B S G O O E I X T B S O K R Q N O R G H T L A A E B H
B X R I M X E I I U D W E E N H C E E Z T E D E G E P J C P M N B O A
W I X I B L K I I U D W E E N H C E E X Q F H T N Y L U A M A G X X L
A J B O I M X F T S N W N A P A I N W R G D U N T E N A O F I I J O A
G I T B P Z A T U C G F B O N A G I W W G Q W Q T O E O T W S E C U E Z
Y C Y F H H I F G M V S U H T P S Q R T O E O E I V R I X B C Y V I I
E X Q T W A M E N E I V L I I A P A D Z C O K L I M R A I C E U Z O O
S L L A T D R A W O T R O L L A T Z V Z C O K L I M R A I C A M L K X
D O N T O E F R L L I K O T O G R O W T H I N S C C C H I C A S B K Z
```

☐ WHAT IS GIVEN
☐ ONE/TENTH (1/10)
☐ -FORM
☐ CAVITY
☐ ANTI-
☐ ECTO-
☐ PAIN
☐ CAUS-
☐ BASIC
☐ ENEMA
☐ MILK
☐ ACOUST/I-
☐ DON'T/O-
☐ APART OR UP
☐ SHARP
☐ TO CLUMP

☐ TO KILL
☐ GANGLI/O-
☐ CHALAZ/IO-
☐ PAIN
☐ BILE OR GALL
☐ -BLAST
☐ CLOTTING OR CLOT
☐ RGHT
☐ -ARIA
☐ BURN OR HEAT
☐ ERUCT/O-
☐ CONI/O-
☐ COX/A-
☐ UPON
☐ FUND/O-
☐ LITTLE BOX

☐ EXTRA-
☐ AIR OR GAS
☐ -DEFERENS
☐ TALL OR TOWARD TALL
☐ TO GROW THIN
☐ -ERGO
☐ MIXTURE
☐ ACETABUL/O-
☐ JUICE
☐ CENTRO-
☐ FIBUL/O-
☐ ANTR/UM-
☐ CALCO-
☐ DEEP SLEEP
☐ OUTPOUCHING
☐ CRUC/I-

PREFIXES & SUFFIXES Word Search Puzzle

```
Z R A E T N P H B K U F W O L L O H F O E K P H J Q M I H C U S I S O
G Y P O C O R A C O L S Q O H S W L I E J O A Z A A C H I R O U C Y H
Q B R A C Y J K J Y C I A Z V A P F N F C M P O G R T K Y M H A G J J
C D A G R R R E O Y V N G M C R U C B U H I F L P O M O N Q R M N Z R
H Y H D T I C S L N G M C R U C H I F Y H D U S T I E A Q J C I I F T
I K S S N K T E I V Q P I A O B V S I P S S M O D U A C U U A S H S H
L H R A J I P A A G G G L U T N I N O S E J P W N O J S F R C C C K U
O I M L D U P Q Q V J Q P C R S R X C C B C V A I N R S T N E A U I C
F U O O N E K C N U P A G O R Z T O C Y R O E R R I A I E O T R N W J
H F R P K R O I M A R D D A U N G A D E S F T D G M C O G I A R P W P
A S B E S T O S D I S L O C A T I O N O Y T I U U U H U R N B Y T J M
W K R C B O K A C P U K A R G A Z U M P O Y O L L B M K O M U I U Q R
C H E I L O Y B K C W N I O D M V C S A E G S O W L S R F A L N O V T
S E C T O Q U I V E R G V F G Z N A U Y V W B V Z A S H O H O G P S U
M E X C I S I O O R R E M O V A L J K L I J O I N T T B L W F J W K L
```

☐ CERBR/O-
☐ DISLOCATION
☐ -CUSIS
☐ PELVIS
☐ EXCISIO OR REMOVAL
☐ ASBEST/O-
☐ CORAC/O-
☐ CRYO-
☐ CYSTIDO-
☐ TEAR
☐ HOLLOW
☐ ALBUMIN/O-
☐ JOINT
☐ WORM
☐ MISCARRYING
☐ OUTPOUCHING
☐ HUMAN

☐ AGGGLUTNIN/O-
☐ AMPHI-
☐ CHIRO-
☐ FIRST
☐ CAUD/O-
☐ -AGRA
☐ CYST-
☐ -CRIT
☐ ETI/O-
☐ TOWARD
☐ HARD
☐ KENO-
☐ AMNIO-
☐ CHILO-
☐ CHEIL/O-
☐ DUST
☐ GRINDING

☐ -CLYSIS
☐ GOOD OR NORMAL
☐ SHARP
☐ ALOPEC/I-
☐ ARTICUL/O-
☐ ACCESS/O-
☐ SCAR
☐ CULD/O-
☐ CUPS
☐ FORGETFUL
☐ ACETABUL/O-
☐ BASIC
☐ PAIN
☐ FEC/O-
☐ TO QUIVER
☐ SKIN

PREFIXES & SUFFIXES Matching

Write the code corresponding to the correct match in the space provided.

___ 1. dactylo-	A1. eyelash or eyelash like
___ 2. concuss/i-	B1. rib
___ 3. -agra	C1. empty or common
___ 4. duoden/o-	D1. green
___ 5. alveol/i-	E1. elbow
___ 6. chlor/o-	F1. egg white
___ 7. acrachn/	G1. skin
___ 8. aggglutnin/o-	H1. breakdown
___ 9. cal/o-	I1. refers to or action
___ 10. caput-	J1. outside, outward, outer or out
___ 11. alopec/i-	K1. head
___ 12. ef-	L1. pubic region
___ 13. enamel	M1. to marry, unite, or sexual union
___ 14. faci/o-	N1. breakdown or down
___ 15. clavicul/o-	O1. juice out
___ 16. -cid	P1. whip
___ 17. dia-	Q1. to blow
___ 18. bulba-	R1. swelling or tumor
___ 19. athero-	S1. heel or lime
___ 20. eczema	T1. eyelid
___ 21. -cusis	U1. cube or cube shaped
___ 22. anter/o-	V1. extremities, height and pointed
___ 23. contra-	W1. work or strength
___ 24. atelo-	X1. cell or chamber
___ 25. -ergo	Y1. pain
___ 26. amblyo-	Z1. without or lack of
___ 27. -DESIS	A2. burn or heat
___ 28. con-	B2. to flow
___ 29. emphysema	C2. rounding
___ 30. dextr/o-	D2. work or labor
___ 31. blenno-	E2. two
___ 32. -enchyma	F2. to kill
___ 33. ceru-	G2. window
___ 34. Beri-	H2. receiver
___ 35. epi-	I2. SKIN
___ 36. cav-	J2. bister or vesicle

____ 37. doct/o-

____ 38. cord-

____ 39. anthrac/o-

____ 40. -cept-

____ 41. cub/o-

____ 42. dacryo-

____ 43. galact/o-

____ 44. convolo-

____ 45. dolich/o-

____ 46. sterco-

____ 47. cleido-

____ 48. cell/o-

____ 49. carbuncul/o-

____ 50. chorea-

____ 51. colob/o-

____ 52. chole-

____ 53. emmetr/o-

____ 54. cimex-

____ 55. attrit/i-

____ 56. chondr/o-

____ 57. fila-

____ 58. doch/o-

____ 59. -emesis

____ 60. comato-

____ 61. eccrine-

____ 62. cebo-

____ 63. alb/o-

____ 64. -ar

____ 65. fibro-

____ 66. fimbri/o-

____ 67. -ectomy

____ 68. e-

____ 69. arche/o-

____ 70. bronch/i-

____ 71. append/o-

____ 72. chancr/o-

____ 73. antr/o-

____ 74. canth/o-

____ 75. ec-

____ 76. cryo-

K2. refers to

L2. wearing out

M2. appendage

N2. cavity

O2. to separate or apart

P2. small

Q2. pipe or pipe-stem

R2. weakness

S2. to separate or apart

T2. gland

U2. cavity or cavern

V2. across, through, total or complete, or between

W2. anything poured in (essential organ part)

X2. out, outside, outward

Y2. diseased or bad

Z2. without or lack of

A3. unequal

B3. burn or heat

C3. cups

D3. face

E3. process of or procedure of

F3. breakdown

G3. blister or vesicle

H3. coal or carbuncle

I3. sac, wine-sac, or pouch

J3. leg thigh or femur

K3. branch or fork

L3. a giving

M3. glowing white

N3. before

O3. ROD-LIKE

P3. flowing

Q3. separate

R3. axle or axis

S3. swelling

T3. to flee

U3. gallbladder

V3. axle or axis

W3. to miscarry or miscarrying (natural or induced)

X3. relaxation

___ 77. acetabul/o-	Y3. glowing ember
___ 78. front/o-	Z3. glowing ember
___ 79. azoto-	A4. empty or common
___ 80. antr/um-	B4. process of or procedure of
___ 81. facet	C4. leg thigh or femur
___ 82. axio-	D4. colon big or large intestine
___ 83. abrupt/io-	E4. back
___ 84. digit-	F4. what is given
___ 85. gangli/o-	G4. glue
___ 86. episi/o-	H4. sun, ray, radium
___ 87. com-	I4. to carry
___ 88. amino-	J4. pain
___ 89. -cytosis	K4. out or remove
___ 90. contrecoup	L4. hook, clavicle or collar bone
___ 91. desmo-	M4. shaped shape or form
___ 92. eosin/o-	N4. twelve
___ 93. azygo-	O4. opening
___ 94. calix-	P4. cut or to cut
___ 95. cycl/o-	Q4. out, outside, outward
___ 96. atri/o-	R4. coal or carbuncle
___ 97. ect-	S4. bent
___ 98. arachino-	T4. worm
___ 99. encephal/o-	U4. carbon dioxide
___ 100. anil/i-	V4. red
___ 101. diplo-	W4. outside, outward, outer or out
___ 102. demi-	X4. dilation
___ 103. centi-	Y4. crab-like
___ 104. ecchymo/-	Z4. bile duct
___ 105. en-	A5. colon big or large intestine
___ 106. adip/o-	B5. against
___ 107. crus/o-	C5. fuse or bind
___ 108. cistern/o-	D5. counter blow
___ 109. asthma-	E5. capable of
___ 110. anti-	F5. boil
___ 111. brach/i-	G5. lip
___ 112. chrom/o-	H5. mushroom
___ 113. culd/o-	I5. above or upon
___ 114. debride-	J5. secret
___ 115. acus-	K5. life
___ 116. -aria	L5. red or flushed
___ 117. conjuctiv/o-	M5. increase (in number)

___ 118. -al	N5. to marry, unite, or sexual union
___ 119. gangren/o-	O5. abdomen or belly
___ 120. du/o-	P5. ROD
___ 121. chalas/i-	Q5. neck
___ 122. ambul/o-	R5. self
___ 123. brady-	S5. hearing
___ 124. fulv/o-	T5. freeze or congeal
___ 125. coel-	U5. belching
___ 126. chalaz/io-	V5. to teach or teacher
___ 127. bula-	W5. first
___ 128. cox/a-	X5. skull
___ 129. fibul/o-	Y5. dilation or ballooning
___ 130. fulgur/o-	Z5. navel
___ 131. -clalasia	A6. spider
___ 132. chordo- (cordo-)	B6. human
___ 133. entero-	C6. bile or gall
___ 134. enema	D6. pain
___ 135. avuls/i-	E6. juice
___ 136. calcane/o-	F6. away
___ 137. cardi/o-	G6. dust
___ 138. caust/o-	H6. TOOTH OR TEETH
___ 139. fet/o-	I6. to nourish
___ 140. delta	J6. scab
___ 141. crypto-	K6. surgical puncture to drain fluid
___ 142. eu-	L6. center
___ 143. acu-	M6. tear
___ 144. -amine	N6. kind
___ 145. -blast	O6. farther from
___ 146. capsulo-	P6. cause
___ 147. chyle-	Q6. spider
___ 148. anxio-	R6. pebbles or granules (of calcium mineral)
___ 149. -us	S6. half
___ 150. currett/o-	T6. pain
___ 151. ar-	U6. to listen
___ 152. carcin/o-	V6. cheek
___ 153. flex-	W6. thread
___ 154. access/o-	X6. prickly, spiny or notched
___ 155. -ation	Y6. jointed
___ 156. dos/e- (dose)	Z6. testis or teste
___ 157. -ate	A7. hand

___ 158. an/o-	B7. hollow belly (cavity)
___ 159. cine/o-	C7. chambers
___ 160. cheil/o-	D7. ulcer (sore)
___ 161. arteri/o-	E7. head
___ 162. bleb/o- (bulla-)	F7. incomplete, without end, imperfect (ending)
___ 163. cirrh/o-	G7. one who
___ 164. capit/o-	H7. iron
___ 165. decem-	I7. digits (fingers and toes)
___ 166. endo-	J7. diffucult, faulty or painful
___ 167. amylo-	K7. LOWER
___ 168. adhes/io-	L7. removal
___ 169. acne	M7. puffed up
___ 170. crenat/o-	N7. milk
___ 171. dys-	O7. calcium
___ 172. chyme-	P7. hip, hip joint, (pelvis and femur)
___ 173. caud/o-	Q7. good or normal
___ 174. cac/o-	R7. fiber
___ 175. -ference	S7. single
___ 176. -crin	T7. horn or horny
___ 177. -continence	U7. toward
___ 178. aspergill/o-	V7. weakness
___ 179. coron/o-	W7. rght
___ 180. ascar/i-	X7. two
___ 181. fibrin/o-	Y7. thread
___ 182. aut-	Z7. upon
___ 183. ancone-	A8. twisted
___ 184. cras/o-	B8. relates to or pertains to
___ 185. aden/o-	C8. excessive sweating
___ 186. angin/o-	D8. secreting or to secrete
___ 187. cellul/o-	E8. heat, heated or hot
___ 188. -asthenia	F8. both
___ 189. abdomin/o-	G8. hard
___ 190. cochle/o-	H8. clotting or clot
___ 191. cyst/o-	I8. hardened skin
___ 192. coagulo/o-	J8. blue
___ 193. -crine	K8. tree-shaped
___ 194. circum-	L8. cornea or horn (shape)
___ 195. effus-	M8. lesser or smaller
___ 196. coni/o-	N8. to bend
___ 197. dura-	O8. hard
___ 198. corne/o-	P8. bug

___ 199. -dynia	Q8. abnormal
___ 200. diaphoro-	R8. without expansion or dilation
___ 201. cyan/o-	S8. thigh
___ 202. caus-	T8. notched
___ 203. an-	U8. old women
___ 204. eti/o-	V8. brown
___ 205. crur/o-	W8. to come together (sexual union; inter/course "between/a flowing")
___ 206. anis/o-	X8. ring
___ 207. aster/o-	Y8. walls
___ 208. cil/i-	Z8. movement filming
___ 209. auscult/o-	A9. instrument
___ 210. fossa-	B9. shell
___ 211. edema-	C9. intestine (usually refers to small intestine)
___ 212. Bin-	D9. thread
___ 213. chiro-	E9. young
___ 214. DON'T/O-	F9. knot swelling or collection knot
___ 215. -cicatrix	G9. blind pouch
___ 216. brux-	H9. dilation
___ 217. febr/o-	I9. good or normal
___ 218. anuerysm-	J9. vagina
___ 219. cyth-	K9. lambs caul 'small cap'
___ 220. -didymis	L9. bladder or sac
___ 221. abcess	M9. little box
___ 222. asco-	N9. eyelash-like
___ 223. -flect	O9. man or male
___ 224. fiss-	P9. hard
___ 225. Balan/o-	Q9. to let down into
___ 226. -ectasis	R9. pain
___ 227. -cis	S9. heart
___ 228. fenestr/o-	T9. hearing
___ 229. cutis-	U9. refers to
___ 230. amnesi/o-	V9. panting
___ 231. ankyl/o-	W9. eating sore
___ 232. keno-	X9. scar
___ 233. cerbr/o-	Y9. within head brain
___ 234. cubit/o-	Z9. furrow or shallow depression
___ 235. echo-	A10. most inward
___ 236. flagell/o-	B10. to clasp
___ 237. atm/o-	C10. crowning
___ 238. cata-	D10. two

___ 239. -agon

___ 240. cholecyst/o-

___ 241. colla/o-

___ 242. bol/o-

___ 243. exo-

___ 244. -artresia

___ 245. deuter/o-

___ 246. ecto-

___ 247. Bacteri/o-

___ 248. bulimo-

___ 249. call/o-

___ 250. fund/o-

___ 251. alges/i-

___ 252. candid/i-

___ 253. DERM/O-

___ 254. foc/o-

___ 255. flat/o-

___ 256. acr/o-

___ 257. fibrill/o-

___ 258. brucca-

___ 259. axill/o-

___ 260. carp/o-

___ 261. dwarf/o-

___ 262. cec/o-

___ 263. colpo-

___ 264. ab-

___ 265. dromo-

___ 266. -eal

___ 267. -conis

___ 268. estr/o-

___ 269. crust/-

___ 270. arthr/o-

___ 271. cholangio-

___ 272. dy/o-

___ 273. apo-

___ 274. dist/o-

___ 275. deca-

___ 276. cephalo-

___ 277. flu-

___ 278. cruc/i-

___ 279. fac-

E10. ear

F10. SKIN

G10. beginning or young

H10. supplemental

I10. center

J10. blood

K10. fat

L10. body

M10. early

N10. a going away

O10. face

P10. cartilage

Q10. HEAVY

R10. little dragon (worm)

S10. refers to or pertains to

T10. chamber

U10. circle

V10. injection

W10. vomit

X10. hair-like

Y10. air or gas

Z10. collar bone (little key shape)

A11. scooping or scraping

B11. basic

C11. air

D11. to stick (together)

E11. to clump

F11. to cloak or cover

G11. to mutilate

H11. cause

I11. bladder or sac

J11. cross or cross-like

K11. snail-like

L11. to boil out

M11. making

N11. to roll together

O11. long, seperation, dislocation

P11. hailstone (eyelid sebaceous cyst)

Q11. to grow thin

R11. star

S11. little fountain

____ 280. ceno-

____ 281. -er

____ 282. asbest/o-

____ 283. af-

____ 284. gamet/o-

____ 285. di-

____ 286. cataract

____ 287. diverticul/o-

____ 288. DEPRESS-

____ 289. brachy-

____ 290. cune/i-

____ 291. -cece

____ 292. gastr/o-

____ 293. gelat/o-

____ 294. eschar

____ 295. -clas

____ 296. corac/o-

____ 297. arche-

____ 298. Bil/i- (bil-)

____ 299. fili-

____ 300. cili-

____ 301. amphi-

____ 302. Bacill/o

____ 303. different-

____ 304. aponeur/o-

____ 305. de-

____ 306. cori/o-

____ 307. carbun/o-

____ 308. cholera-

____ 309. Bas/o-

____ 310. erythermat/o-

____ 311. catheter/o-

____ 312. -clysis

____ 313. cuti/o- (cut-)

____ 314. -deferens

____ 315. bio-

____ 316. -dote

____ 317. calcin/o-

____ 318. fec/o-

____ 319. capn/o-

T11. starch

U11. one/tenth (1/10)

V11. band

W11. corner of eye

X11. normal or correct

Y11. knuckle (nob)

Z11. cavity

A12. to split or splitting

B12. one who

C12. cold

D12. both

E12. forehead or before

F12. near or beside

G12. finger or toe

H12. soft

I12. together

J12. at a base

K12. wrist

L12. out, outside, outward

M12. crowning frontal body cut

N12. windpipe or tracea-like

O12. water

P12. away from or reversed

Q12. lump or ball

R12. to bend

S12. srool, fecal matter or dung

T12. vapor or steam

U12. mucus

V12. heel

W12. together joined (united)

X12. to void (expel) urine

Y12. restlessness, uneasy, apprehensive

Z12. to tear

A13. porridge or yellow fat

B13. dim vision

C13. grinding

D13. away or out

E13. inducing or leading

F13. within or inside

G13. ring

____ 320. -able
____ 321. filar/i-
____ 322. dis-
____ 323. capill/o-
____ 324. fontan/o-
____ 325. cric/o-
____ 326. acoust/i-
____ 327. dors/o-
____ 328. coit/o-
____ 329. -estasy
____ 330. dendr/o-
____ 331. esthes/i-
____ 332. -ac
____ 333. catarrh-
____ 334. alimento/o
____ 335. chlamyd/i-
____ 336. anthr/o-
____ 337. echin/o-
____ 338. calco-
____ 339. aqua-
____ 340. -cyesis
____ 341. furc/o-
____ 342. cerv/i-
____ 343. dracuncul/o-
____ 344. -cele
____ 345. -ellum
____ 346. ex-
____ 347. gelatino-
____ 348. ad-
____ 349. erthr/o-
____ 350. condyl/o-
____ 351. eruct/o-
____ 352. colon/o-
____ 353. caligi/o-
____ 354. anecto-
____ 355. anomal/y
____ 356. auricul/o-
____ 357. enuresis-
____ 358. -fuge
____ 359. Bi-
____ 360. Benign/i-

H13. lip
I13. upon tendon (sheet or sheath around tendon)
J13. sound
K13. short
L13. skin
M13. irrigation or injection
N13. organic compound
O13. fox mange or baldness
P13. fiber-like
Q13. PENIS (GLANS PENIS)
R13. two or a pair
S13. blister
T13. refers to or pertains to
U13. to quiver
V13. stool, fecal matter, or dung
W13. rose red (color)
X13. bladder or sac
Y13. hollow
Z13. pointed
A14. lack of or without
B14. away (away from)
C14. excisio or removal
D14. thread
E14. hunger
F14. berry
G14. billary acute diarrhea
H14. head
I14. juice
J14. in
K14. fleshy or flesh
L14. orgasm
M14. sieve
N14. to sprinkle
O14. tailbone
P14. mixture
Q14. relaxation
R14. skin
S14. before or foremost (in front)
T14. blind pouch
U14. cone shaped
V14. away or out

___ 361. deka-, dek-	W14. tall or toward tall
___ 362. cau-	X14. little
___ 363. Bary-	Y14. sharp
___ 364. DERMAT/O-	Z14. bag
___ 365. -e	A15. base or lage part (organ body)
___ 366. chiasma	B15. secrete
___ 367. -form	C15. turmoil
___ 368. -creas	D15. fan shaped or triangular
___ 369. acanth/o-	E15. gallbladder duct (canal)
___ 370. auto-	F15. one-hundredth apart
___ 371. calyx-	G15. toward
___ 372. core/o-	H15. to tear away from
___ 373. crani/o-	I15. bladder or sac
___ 374. carb/o-	J15. enzyme
___ 375. cement/o-	K15. TOOTH OR TEETH
___ 376. dol/o-	L15. bile or gall (ingredient of)
___ 377. audi-	M15. two
___ 378. -borg	N15. armpit or central
___ 379. dipther/i-	O15. outside, outward, outer or out
___ 380. cost/o-	P15. outpouching
___ 381. andr/o-	Q15. before
___ 382. conch/a-	R15. arm
___ 383. centr/i-	S15. to walk
___ 384. cusp/i-	T15. to flow down
___ 385. fract/o-	U15. joint
___ 386. cyte-	V15. ten
___ 387. coronal plane (aka: frontal plane)	W15. nitrogen compound
___ 388. fasc/i-	X15. hip, hip joint, (pelvis and femur)
___ 389. clon/o-	Y15. refers to
___ 390. corp/o-	Z15. burn or heat
___ 391. calx-	A16. to draw or to lead (motion) away
___ 392. angi/o-	B16. double or two
___ 393. cornu-	C16. cord
___ 394. aer/o-	D16. fever
___ 395. ethm/o-	E16. freeze or congeal
___ 396. cyst-	F16. belly
___ 397. Bene-	G16. feeling (physical)
___ 398. electr/o-	H16. pupil or iris (rainbow)
___ 399. anthrop/o-	I16. self
___ 400. Bas/io-	J16. short

____ 401. cyst/i-
____ 402. furun/o-
____ 403. ernia
____ 404. -facient
____ 405. gam/o-
____ 406. embryo-
____ 407. cyt-
____ 408. DENT/O-
____ 409. burs/o-
____ 410. duct/o-
____ 411. eso-
____ 412. fistul/o-
____ 413. choledoch/o-
____ 414. coccyg/o-
____ 415. femor/o-
____ 416. eti/o-
____ 417. dem/o-
____ 418. amnio-
____ 419. dynam/o-
____ 420. fore-
____ 421. -age
____ 422. aur/i-
____ 423. -clast
____ 424. -flux
____ 425. acrom/i-
____ 426. -or
____ 427. -agogue
____ 428. decub/o-
____ 429. -algia
____ 430. em-
____ 431. clubb/o-
____ 432. extra-
____ 433. brevi-
____ 434. flacci/o-
____ 435. -cule
____ 436. axo-
____ 437. ambi-
____ 438. actin/o-
____ 439. emac/i-
____ 440. col/o-
____ 441. -crit

K16. to lighten (with sparks burning tissue)
L16. stool, fecal matter, or dung
M16. violent shaking
N16. bruise
O16. wax
P16. urea nitrogen
Q16. to choke
R16. around
S16. contained
T16. meal or food
U16. secrete
V16. refers to or pertains to
W16. extremities, height and pointed
X16. crows beak (shape)
Y16. vinegar cup or hip joint (for femur)
Z16. vessel
A17. one/tenth (1/10)
B17. thirst or thirsty
C17. WEIGHT
D17. ear
E17. colored
F17. scab or outer coat
G17. a crossing
H17. two
I17. second or secondary
J17. bark, outer bark, rind, or cortex
K17. first
L17. dancing (shaking)
M17. cell or chamber
N17. white
O17. stomach
P17. face
Q17. sharp
R17. carbon atoms, coal, or charcoal
S17. in
T17. away or out
U17. artery
V17. BINDING, TO BAND OR A BAND
W17. vocal chords cord
X17. pregnancy
Y17. hearing

____ 442. blepharo- (palpebro-)
____ 443. centro-
____ 444. cystido-
____ 445. -apheresis
____ 446. ante-
____ 447. albumin/o-
____ 448. articul/o-
____ 449. scato-
____ 450. contus/i-
____ 451. dips/o-
____ 452. co-
____ 453. -ase
____ 454. ferro-
____ 455. -collis
____ 456. Baro-
____ 457. -ition
____ 458. fil-
____ 459. clino-
____ 460. ana-
____ 461. formamen/o-
____ 462. chilo-
____ 463. deep
____ 464. fungi-
____ 465. -ory
____ 466. -coccus
____ 467. cox/o-
____ 468. -ary
____ 469. abort/io
____ 470. cortic/o-
____ 471. effer-
____ 472. a-
____ 473. -centesis

Z17. unquenchable
A18. waterfall or cloudiness
B18. brain
C18. electrical
D18. apart or up
E18. cavity
F18. to lie down
G18. dull
H18. female
I18. yellow-oranged (jaundiced)
J18. refers to
K18. slow
L18. to break
M18. center or hearth
N18. forgetful
O18. fingers
P18. elbow
Q18. wedge
R18. closure
S18. to remove or separate
T18. cell or chamber
U18. ligament (also tendon)
V18. thorny (skin growth)
W18. cups
X18. deep sleep
Y18. running
Z18. against
A19. together
B19. people
C19. pointed
D19. membrane
E19. duct or canal

PREFIXES & SUFFIXES Quiz

Circle the letter of the Meaning that corresponds to the displayed Prefix/Suffix.

1. ef-

    A. pain

    B. colon big or large intestine

    C. to draw or to lead (motion) away

    D. away or out

2. azoto-

    A. to cloak or cover

    B. secret

    C. urea nitrogen

    D. carbon dioxide

3. -ference

    A. corner of eye

    B. to carry

    C. cube or cube shaped

    D. head

4. fungi-

    A. extremities, height and pointed

    B. apart or up

    C. mushroom

    D. ROD-LIKE

5. digit-

    A. wearing out

    B. ulcer (sore)

    C. finger or toe

    D. cell or chamber

6. ceru-

    A. to flow

    B. cheek

    C. wax

    D. cups

7. deuter/o-

A. second or secondary

B. yellow-oranged (jaundiced)

C. to draw or to lead (motion) away

D. fuse or bind

8. -deferens

A. freeze or congeal

B. to separate or apart

C. opening

D. bile or gall

9. alges/i-

A. pain

B. extremities, height and pointed

C. WEIGHT

D. porridge or yellow fat

10. cyte-

A. short

B. gallbladder duct (canal)

C. twelve

D. cell or chamber

Circle the letter of the Prefix/Suffix that corresponds to the displayed Meaning.

11. apart or up

A. debride-

B. anxio-

C. fec/o-

D. ana-

12. gallbladder

A. cholecyst/o-

B. contus/i-

C. fila-

D. cau-

13. stool, fecal matter, or dung

A. dacryo-

B. formamen/o-

C. burs/o-

D. scato-

14. heat, heated or hot

    A. gam/o-

    B. -flect

    C. cutis-

    D. cal/o-

15. cavity

    A. -cusis

    B. cistern/o-

    C. cortic/o-

    D. comato-

16. eating sore

    A. gangren/o-

    B. cras/o-

    C. dactylo-

    D. effer-

17. to lighten (with sparks burning tissue)

    A. bulimo-

    B. ante-

    C. dynam/o-

    D. fulgur/o-

18. to bend

    A. choledoch/o-

    B. -flect

    C. asbest/o-

    D. cystido-

19. air

    A. corne/o-

    B. -aria

    C. deep

    D. crus/o-

20. water

    A. foc/o-

    B. aqua-

    C. -flect

    D. aur/i-

21. process of or procedure of

PREFIXES & SUFFIXES Quiz

Circle the letter of the Meaning that corresponds to the displayed Prefix/Suffix.

1. cac/o-

    A. meal or food

    B. face

    C. empty or common

    D. diseased or bad

2. cebo-

    A. meal or food

    B. burn or heat

    C. vagina

    D. thorny (skin growth)

3. fiss-

    A. hearing

    B. to split or splitting

    C. process of or procedure of

    D. bladder or sac

4. gelat/o-

    A. freeze or congeal

    B. axle or axis

    C. kind

    D. injection

5. -enchyma

    A. two

    B. anything poured in (essential organ part)

    C. thread

    D. secrete

6. -estasy

    A. panting

    B. fingers

    C. empty or common

    D. dilation

7. flu-

A. flowing

B. circle

C. to carry

D. relaxation

8. delta

A. beginning or young

B. hard

C. fan shaped or triangular

D. to listen

9. acus-

A. near or beside

B. face

C. fox mange or baldness

D. sharp

10. ethm/o-

A. thread

B. dilation

C. sieve

D. skull

Circle the letter of the Prefix/Suffix that corresponds to the displayed Meaning.

11. cartilage

A. crus/o-

B. chondr/o-

C. convolo-

D. fenestr/o-

12. skull

A. gangli/o-

B. coronal plane (aka: frontal plane)

C. crani/o-

D. fract/o-

13. bile or gall

A. Bil/i- (bil-)

B. -ellum

C. abrupt/io-

D. -cytosis

14. gallbladder

    A. cholecyst/o-

    B. gamet/o-

    C. ef-

    D. capit/o-

15. hair-like

    A. emphysema

    B. gangren/o-

    C. capill/o-

    D. acrachn/

16. forgetful

    A. dors/o-

    B. amnesi/o-

    C. extra-

    D. -flect

17. water

    A. Bas/io-

    B. deka-, dek-

    C. aqua-

    D. -facient

18. cheek

    A. carbuncul/o-

    B. gangli/o-

    C. amnesi/o-

    D. brucca-

19. heat, heated or hot

    A. -cusis

    B. cal/o-

    C. aponeur/o-

    D. facet

20. star

    A. aster/o-

    B. cyst/o-

    C. fund/o-

    D. ceno-

EXTRA CREDIT: Give the Prefix/Suffix that corresponds to the displayed Meaning.

21. window

PREFIXES & SUFFIXES Quiz

Circle the letter of the Meaning that corresponds to the displayed Prefix/Suffix.

1. azoto-
    A. to mutilate
    B. eyelash or eyelash like
    C. urea nitrogen
    D. to choke

2. flex-
    A. weakness
    B. instrument
    C. to bend
    D. empty or common

3. -agogue
    A. inducing or leading
    B. injection
    C. out, outside, outward
    D. gallbladder

4. -cept-
    A. heel or lime
    B. scar
    C. cube or cube shaped
    D. receiver

5. crus/o-
    A. neck
    B. pain
    C. ear
    D. leg thigh or femur

6. cell/o-
    A. away (away from)
    B. abdomen or belly
    C. to boil out
    D. slow

7. dactylo-

A. sound

B. digits (fingers and toes)

C. lip

D. brown

8. auricul/o-

A. single

B. stool, fecal matter, or dung

C. ear

D. tailbone

9. diaphoro-

A. cheek

B. excessive sweating

C. unequal

D. together

10. sterco-

A. increase (in number)

B. srool, fecal matter or dung

C. whip

D. bladder or sac

Circle the letter of the Prefix/Suffix that corresponds to the displayed Meaning.

11. together joined (united)

A. bulba-

B. conjuctiv/o-

C. ec-

D. cystido-

12. to cloak or cover

A. cortic/o-

B. flat/o-

C. carbun/o-

D. chlamyd/i-

13. to separate or apart

A. different-

B. deca-

C. amnio-

D. albumin/o-

14. eyelid

    A. blepharo- (palpebro-)
    B. -cept-
    C. eschar
    D. bula-

15. short

    A. brachy-
    B. ana-
    C. diplo-
    D. chancr/o-

16. finger or toe

    A. flacci/o-
    B. digit-
    C. corp/o-
    D. culd/o-

17. skin

    A. comato-
    B. flacci/o-
    C. cori/o-
    D. femor/o-

18. freeze or congeal

    A. gelatino-
    B. dura-
    C. carb/o-
    D. cuti/o- (cut-)

19. starch

    A. access/o-
    B. auscult/o-
    C. amylo-
    D. cephalo-

20. waterfall or cloudiness

    A. cataract
    B. cori/o-
    C. articul/o-
    D. asbest/o-

EXTRA CREDIT: Give the Prefix/Suffix that corresponds to the displayed Meaning.

21. deep sleep

PREFIXES & SUFFIXES Quiz

Circle the letter of the Meaning that corresponds to the displayed Prefix/Suffix.

1. cyst/i-
   - A. to carry
   - B. bladder or sac
   - C. prickly, spiny or notched
   - D. fat

2. fiss-
   - A. to split or splitting
   - B. before or foremost (in front)
   - C. tree-shaped
   - D. two

3. cal/o-
   - A. heat, heated or hot
   - B. most inward
   - C. two or a pair
   - D. ulcer (sore)

4. chilo-
   - A. ear
   - B. fleshy or flesh
   - C. spider
   - D. lip

5. eti/o-
   - A. to lighten (with sparks burning tissue)
   - B. dilation or ballooning
   - C. one/tenth (1/10)
   - D. cause

6. blenno-
   - A. mucus
   - B. single
   - C. waterfall or cloudiness
   - D. long, seperation, dislocation

7. flu-

A. around

B. flowing

C. single

D. above or upon

8. cellul/o-

A. skin

B. outpouching

C. chambers

D. notched

9. -estasy

A. dilation

B. outside, outward, outer or out

C. ring

D. boil

10. cruc/i-

A. eyelid

B. intestine (usually refers to small intestine)

C. enzyme

D. cross or cross-like

Circle the letter of the Prefix/Suffix that corresponds to the displayed Meaning.

11. burn or heat

A. circum-

B. cau-

C. an-

D. ankyl/o-

12. both

A. ambi-

B. ankyl/o-

C. centr/i-

D. cutis-

13. hollow belly (cavity)

A. fossa-

B. arche-

C. chyle-

D. coel-

14. running
   A. cata-
   B. dromo-
   C. calix-
   D. an-

15. to blow
   A. dis-
   B. flat/o-
   C. anthr/o-
   D. dia-

16. empty or common
   A. -DESIS
   B. ceno-
   C. corp/o-
   D. -ectomy

17. a crossing
   A. chiasma
   B. cornu-
   C. -dynia
   D. -deferens

18. movement filming
   A. cori/o-
   B. -conis
   C. azoto-
   D. cine/o-

19. iron
   A. cornu-
   B. extra-
   C. caust/o-
   D. ferro-

20. to kill
   A. -cid
   B. anthrac/o-
   C. em-
   D. centro-

21. diseased or bad

PREFIXES & SUFFIXES Quiz

Circle the letter of the Meaning that corresponds to the displayed Prefix/Suffix.

1. -asthenia

    A. head

    B. self

    C. weakness

    D. away or out

2. cori/o-

    A. ring

    B. cheek

    C. skin

    D. thirst or thirsty

3. aden/o-

    A. gland

    B. in

    C. crows beak (shape)

    D. panting

4. dys-

    A. skin

    B. diffucult, faulty or painful

    C. puffed up

    D. ligament (also tendon)

5. flex-

    A. fan shaped or triangular

    B. scar

    C. slow

    D. to bend

6. clubb/o-

    A. cone shaped

    B. notched

    C. rounding

    D. mixture

7. abdomin/o-

A. yellow-oranged (jaundiced)

B. ROD-LIKE

C. to listen

D. belly

8. -able

A. together joined (united)

B. green

C. capable of

D. within or inside

9. fila-

A. panting

B. cavity

C. thread

D. scooping or scraping

10. -cusis

A. to quiver

B. hearing

C. away (away from)

D. both

Circle the letter of the Prefix/Suffix that corresponds to the displayed Meaning.

11. stool, fecal matter, or dung

A. scato-

B. caust/o-

C. chordo- (cordo-)

D. -cis

12. hunger

A. digit-

B. bulim o-

C. eti/o-

D. asbest/o-

13. axle or axis

A. Bene-

B. axio-

C. aqua-

D. crust/-

14. double or two
    A. cox/o-
    B. em-
    C. diplo-
    D. Benign/i-

15. short
    A. brevi-
    B. gangren/o-
    C. cerbr/o-
    D. condyl/o-

16. face
    A. coel-
    B. fac-
    C. -or
    D. -er

17. TOOTH OR TEETH
    A. bulba-
    B. -agra
    C. alveol/i-
    D. DENT/O-

18. most inward
    A. -clysis
    B. crani/o-
    C. calx-
    D. deep

19. dilation or ballooning
    A. culd/o-
    B. caus-
    C. anuerysm-
    D. -form

20. to tear
    A. -didymis
    B. fund/o-
    C. anthrop/o-
    D. avuls/i-

EXTRA CREDIT: Give the Meaning that corresponds to the displayed Prefix/Suffix.

21. chyle-

PREFIXES & SUFFIXES Test

Enter the letter for the matching Meaning

1. ☐ Baro-
2. ☐ echo-
3. ☐ ceno-
4. ☐ andr/o-
5. ☐ cyte-
6. ☐ af-
7. ☐ erythermat/o-
8. ☐ cellul/o-
9. ☐ bio-
10. ☐ diverticul/o-
11. ☐ blenno-
12. ☐ en-
13. ☐ fulgur/o-
14. ☐ cori/o-
15. ☐ centr/i-
16. ☐ eu-
17. ☐ -continence
18. ☐ bol/o-
19. ☐ gangren/o-
20. ☐ edema-

A. eating sore
B. man or male
C. toward
D. lump or ball
E. center
F. chambers
G. contained
H. WEIGHT
I. empty or common
J. mucus
K. outpouching
L. life
M. sound
N. skin
O. good or normal
P. to lighten (with sparks burning tissue)
Q. cell or chamber
R. red or flushed
S. in
T. swelling

Give the Meaning that corresponds to the displayed Prefix/Suffix.

21. anis/o-

22. cerbr/o-

Give the Prefix/Suffix that corresponds to the displayed Meaning.

23. bile or gall (ingredient of)

24.   closure

25.   to blow

26.   iron

27.   to clump

28.   to mutilate

29.   ring

30.   lambs caul 'small cap'

PREFIXES & SUFFIXES Test

Enter the letter for the matching Meaning

1. ☐ contrecoup
2. ☐ alimento/o
3. ☐ centr/i-
4. ☐ cutis-
5. ☐ ecto-
6. ☐ diplo-
7. ☐ centi-
8. ☐ -facient
9. ☐ amnesi/o-
10. ☐ flacci/o-
11. ☐ chalas/i-
12. ☐ concuss/i-
13. ☐ blenno-
14. ☐ chiro-
15. ☐ acanth/o-
16. ☐ abrupt/io-
17. ☐ Bin-
18. ☐ diaphoro-
19. ☐ -centesis
20. ☐ ernia

A. violent shaking
B. to tear away from
C. outside, outward, outer or out
D. to nourish
E. counter blow
F. relaxation
G. surgical puncture to drain fluid
H. skin
I. forgetful
J. thorny (skin growth)
K. center
L. double or two
M. hand
N. two
O. making
P. blood
Q. soft
R. one-hundredth apart
S. mucus
T. excessive sweating

Give the Meaning that corresponds to the displayed Prefix/Suffix.

21. -al

22. effus-

23. dynam/o-

Give the Prefix/Suffix that corresponds to the displayed Meaning.

24. face

25. cups

26. cornea or horn (shape)

27. ear

28. wax

29. sieve

30. stool, fecal matter, or dung

PREFIXES & SUFFIXES Test

Enter the letter for the matching Meaning

1.	☐ coron/o-	A.	stool, fecal matter, or dung
2.	☐ atelo-	B.	forgetful
3.	☐ fec/o-	C.	intestine (usually refers to small intestine)
4.	☐ -able	D.	incomplete, without end, imperfect (ending)
5.	☐ anter/o-	E.	puffed up
6.	☐ decem-	F.	colored
7.	☐ amnesi/o-	G.	two or a pair
8.	☐ crypto-	H.	crowning
9.	☐ chrom/o-	I.	secret
10.	☐ entero-	J.	capable of
11.	☐ centro-	K.	rib
12.	☐ cost/o-	L.	glowing ember
13.	☐ crus/o-	M.	before or foremost (in front)
14.	☐ emphysema	N.	center
15.	☐ fungi-	O.	one/tenth (1/10)
16.	☐ amblyo-	P.	mushroom
17.	☐ dy/o-	Q.	dull
18.	☐ carbun/o-	R.	at a base
19.	☐ Bas/io-	S.	leg thigh or femur
20.	☐ -borg	T.	orgasm

Give the Meaning that corresponds to the displayed Prefix/Suffix.

21. -ary

22. fimbri/o-

23. conch/a-

24.   -conis

Give the Prefix/Suffix that corresponds to the displayed Meaning.

25.   prickly, spiny or notched

26.   abnormal

27.   thread

28.   air

29.   extremities, height and pointed

30.   wedge

PREFIXES & SUFFIXES Test

Enter the letter for the matching Meaning

1.	☐ fund/o-	A.	bug
2.	☐ currett/o-	B.	white
3.	☐ coni/o-	C.	to grow thin
4.	☐ axill/o-	D.	soft
5.	☐ ect-	E.	base or lage part (organ body)
6.	☐ doct/o-	F.	beginning or young
7.	☐ flacci/o-	G.	horn or horny
8.	☐ circum-	H.	feeling (physical)
9.	☐ fibro-	I.	around
10.	☐ access/o-	J.	unequal
11.	☐ alb/o-	K.	coal or carbuncle
12.	☐ -blast	L.	fiber
13.	☐ cimex-	M.	dust
14.	☐ esthes/i-	N.	armpit or central
15.	☐ anthr/o-	O.	refers to or pertains to
16.	☐ cornu-	P.	outside, outward, outer or out
17.	☐ cyst-	Q.	scooping or scraping
18.	☐ -ac	R.	supplemental
19.	☐ emac/i-	S.	to teach or teacher
20.	☐ anis/o-	T.	bladder or sac

Give the Meaning that corresponds to the displayed Prefix/Suffix.

21. culd/o-

22. duoden/o-

23. embryo-

Give the Prefix/Suffix that corresponds to the displayed Meaning.

24. little dragon (worm)

25. ten

26. red

27. ear

28. kind

29. work or labor

30. without expansion or dilation

PREFIXES & SUFFIXES Test

Enter the letter for the matching Meaning

1. ☐ exo-		A.	self
2. ☐ apo-		B.	intestine (usually refers to small intestine)
3. ☐ chrom/o-		C.	out, outside, outward
4. ☐ auto-		D.	weakness
5. ☐ cebo-		E.	to marry, unite, or sexual union
6. ☐ different-		F.	extremities, height and pointed
7. ☐ gamet/o-		G.	above or upon
8. ☐ digit-		H.	to remove or separate
9. ☐ burs/o-		I.	porridge or yellow fat
10. ☐ access/o-		J.	meal or food
11. ☐ crus/o-		K.	supplemental
12. ☐ athero-		L.	colored
13. ☐ entero-		M.	away or out
14. ☐ Beri-		N.	egg white
15. ☐ -apheresis		O.	finger or toe
16. ☐ amnio-		P.	leg thigh or femur
17. ☐ ef-		Q.	to separate or apart
18. ☐ acr/o-		R.	to lie down
19. ☐ decub/o-		S.	sac, wine-sac, or pouch
20. ☐ albumin/o-		T.	lambs caul 'small cap'

Give the Meaning that corresponds to the displayed Prefix/Suffix.

21. dracuncul/o-

22. conjuctiv/o-

23. -ference

24. convolo-

25. doch/o-

Give the Prefix/Suffix that corresponds to the displayed Meaning.

26. human

27. shell

28. process of or procedure of

29. opening

30. cone shaped

www.ingramcontent.com/pod-product-compliance
Lightning Source LLC
Chambersburg PA
CBHW081338160726
48000CB00010B/3145